ACID REFLUX DIET

A Complete Guide to Cook Healthy Food for Healing and Prevent Acid Reflux Disease with Easy Meal Plans and Delicious Recipes, Including Vegan and Gluten-Free

By

Albert Duke

TABLE OF CONTENTS

INTRODUCTION

Congratulations on purchasing *Acid Reflux Diet,* and thank you for doing so.

The following chapters will discuss all of the parts about the Acid Reflux diet that we need to know in order to stop the pain and discomfort and get our health back. There are so many people who suffer from acid reflux, and whether it is something that just happens on occasion or it is a common occurrence, you will find that it is something that needs to be taken care of to keep us healthy. This guidebook is going to take some time to talk about Acid Reflux and what it is doing to our health and some of the basics of what we can do to make it better.

The beginning of this guidebook is going to talk about some of the basics of acid reflux, and what is actually causing the problem in our bodies. Often the issue is not that we have too much acid in the body and the stomach, but that we do not have enough. Getting our body hack into balance is going to be the best way to ensure that we are healthy and that we can take care of our bodies better than before. And one of the best steps to doing this, as we will look at in this guidebook, is through the foods that we eat.

There are a number of topics that we will explain when we are going through this guidebook. We will look at how some of the symptoms that we feel with chronic acid reflux can relate back to the foods that we eat on a regular basis how the battle of the pH could be a big issue here, as with a lot of the other health conditions that we deal with, and some of the simple treatment options, both surgical, medicine related, and natural, that we can utilize in order to get a handle on our acid reflux and make sure that we get it in line.

From there, it is time to get into our eating habits and look more at how the foods we enjoy are going to have a big impact on how we feel. We will spend some time looking at the food lists, which tells us which foods we need to avoid, and which ones we are allowed to have when we follow this diet plan. Then we will look at a meal plan that you can follow that will help you eat the right foods, and avoid the wrong foods, to keep your best health in mind.

Then it is time to get to some of the fun parts of this diet: the recipes. There are so many good options that we are able to use when it is time to worry about our overall health on the acid reflux diet, and you may be surprised at how tasty and good they can be. This guidebook will have some great recipes for breakfast, lunch, snacks dinner, desserts, and even some vegan and vegetarian options, so you always have a lot of variety, and you can take care of your health in no time.

Dealing with acid reflux is not something that anyone of us wants to deal with on a regular basis. It is uncomfortable, and it can be painful, and it does a lot of damage to other parts of our health. When you are ready to get started with the acid reflux diet, and you want to see some of the best results in a short amount of time when it comes to your health, make sure to check out this guidebook to help you get started.

There are plenty of books on this subject on the market, thanks again for choosing this one! Every effort was made to ensure it is full of as much useful information as possible, please enjoy it!

Chapter 1

UNDERSTANDING
YOUR ACID REFLUX

Acid reflux is a serious medical condition that is associated with stomach acid flowing up, which is mostly going to be composed of hydrochloric acid, into the esophagus or the food pipe. In some people, this kind of problem is going to come in between things like burping, which can be embarrassing when it happens in public.

The hydrochloric acid is going to aid in the proper digestion of food and will act as a good protector from bacteria that could form. We have to remember that our stomachs are complex organs that are composed of a lot of different parts. Its lining is designed in order to produce some acid, which will help to digest the food and protect the system against some wear and tear over time, especially when it comes to ulcers that can happen when there is not enough food, and more.

So basically, the acid is supposed to be there. It is there to help us digest our food and to keep the stomach and all of its parts working well. but you will find that there are times when it goes too far and can leave the stomach. When this acid leaves the stomach, it can be dangerous to work with and can cause a lot of damage in the process.

Acid reflux, along with the GERD or gastroesophageal reflux disease, is going to be closely related, even though they are often going to be a little bit different when we work on them. Acid reflux is technically going to be gastroesophageal reflux, and it is when we have a backward flow of the acid in the stomach into the tube that will help to connect our stomachs to our throats, which is known as the esophagus.

During one of the times that we surf from acid reflux, you may feel a kind of burning sensation in your chest, which is going to be heartburn. This can happen when you eat certain foods, when you have a really big meal, or when you have alcohol or coffee. What causes acid reflux is not always the same for each person. Some are able to eat and drink what they want, and others are going to have a lot more troubles and will find that they are more sensitive to this along the way.

Sometimes the acid reflux that we are talking about above will progress into GERD, which is going to be a more severe form of reflux. One of the most common symptoms that we see with the GERD is heartburn, which will show up at least two times a week when you have this kind of condition. Some of the other signs and symptoms that you could have include regurgitation of the food that you eat, a sour liquid that comes up, trouble with swallowing, coughing, chest pain, and wheezing. And these get even worse when you are lying down at night so they can make your sleep schedule go off.

Now, you may find that you have acid reflux on occasion, such as after eating Thanksgiving dinner. This kind, if not really that big of a deal and you should be just fine. But when it becomes a bigger problem, that is when we need to pay attention. And even the occasional type of acid reflux is something that we should pay attention to. If we choose not to, it is possible that the acid reflux is going to get a lot worse, and we could get really sick in the process.

You will find that if you have acid reflux on occasion, then making some lifestyle changes could be the right way to help you out with this. Making sure that you eat meals that are smaller, you lose any of the excess weight that you have, make sure that you are not eating anything a few hours before you plan to go to bed raise your head up when you are sleeping, and then avoid foods that seem to trigger heartburn and you can work on keeping that acid reflux, and all of the damage away.

There are a number of foods that you should be careful about based on how bad the reflux is. Avoiding foods that trigger your heartburn, including fatty or fried foods, and even chocolate and caffeine can ensure that you will not deal with this as much. You should also be careful about wearing clothing that is too tight, especially around your stomach, and avoid having tobacco and alcohol on a regular basis.

If it is necessary, then you may need to work with some medications to help you with your occasional acid reflux. This can include things like taking some antacids, like Tums, or you can take an H-2 receptor blocker to help you get it under control. For most people who deal with the acid reflux just on occasion and not much more, then these are going to work out just fine. But if you are dealing with it on a more frequent basis, then it may be time to make some changes quickly.

If you think that your acid reflux has gone on to the next level and that you are dealing with GERD instead, or you notice that your signs and symptoms are getting worse, you have difficulty with swallowing, vomiting, and nausea. Then it is time to go and talk to your doctor. Doing some lifestyle changes can help with this, but sometimes prescription medications can help you out in the meantime. And in some situations, GERD can be treated with the help of several procedures, including surgery.

Facts Concerning Acid Reflux

There are a lot of different facts that we need to know when it comes to acid reflux and how it behaves in the body. Some of these facts that can help us to better understand what we will discuss in this guidebook, and can prove useful to some of our work along the way include:

1. Acid reflux can come in many names, including gastroesophageal reflux disease, or GERD, or heartburn. Sometimes it will go by the name of pyrosis or acid indigestion.

2. The condition is going to be known as GERD in particular if the symptoms start to show up more than two times a week.

3. It is a very common ailment in the west, and many Americans will suffer from this issue.

4. The esophagus is going to be protected by a part known as the gastroesophageal sphincter, which is going to be composed of muscle, from possible harm from the stomach contents. These muscles need to be in good working order because they are the gate valve that will block the entrance to the stomach.

5. We will experience heartburn when there is some abnormal activity with that sphincter from above. This is because when the sphincter is not working

well, the acid from the stomach could potentially flow up into the food pipe or the esophagus and cause some issues.

6. It is common to notice this one after eating, and some of the symptoms could including burning pain that is below or around the area of the chest.

7. Obesity and smoking are two things that are likely to trigger acid reflux more.

8. It is possible to treat this with some of the over the counter medicines that you may find at the store, and some alternative medicines work well too.

9. It is possible that GERD, if it is left untreated and you do not take care of the issue, can lead to some complications. The complication that is the most feared here is cancer.

10. Heartburn is not going to be related to the heart. It gets this name because the pain that we feel is often going to be below or around the area of the chest.

11. One is sometimes going to notice a sour or a bitter taste in their mouth or throat for a few minutes, and sometimes a few hours with this one.

12. Sleeping with more than one pillow is a good way to get rid of some of the heartburn that you feel.

13. If you spit more often by chewing gum, it can help you to push some of the acids back to the stomach and relieve the pain.

Who is at Risk?

Pretty much anyone can be at risk for dealing with acid reflux, and it is possible that most of us have had it at one time or another. The issue comes into play when we start to deal with the acid reflux on a regular basis, several times a week. It is possible though that this issue can occur at any age and sometimes even children are going to deal with it. There are a few risk factors that can make it more likely that you will have this issue, and those include:

1. If you are fond of lots of salty food.
2. Eating close to bedtime.
3. If you like to eat foods that are spicy or can otherwise irritate the stomach.
4. If your diet is low in fiber.
5. If you have a lifestyle that is mostly sedentary.
6. If you are an active or a passive smoker
7. If you like to wear clothes, pants, and belts that are really tight-fitting.
8. If you are pregnant.
9. If you are obese.

The Complications of Acid Reflux

Having this condition on occasion is not a big deal. It can happen when we eat too much or try something that we know irritates us, but we were out celebrating or having some fun. But when acid reflux happens on a regular basis, it can lead to some big complications if you are not treating it well. both Berrett's esophagus and esophagitis are able to lead to cancer in some patients if it is not treated.

One study that looked at these effects was done in 1999 and is found in the New England Journal of Medicine. The study was able to find the connection between frequent acid reflux and cancer. Patients are then advised to seek medical advice if they notice that the acid reflux is getting worse or if it sticks around even when they are taking medications and applying some home remedies in the process.

There are a lot of issues that can come up with this one. It is possible to deal with Barrett's esophagus, esophagitis, esophageal bleeding, ulcers, esophageal cancer, strictures, and more based on how bad it is, and how long the condition has been going on.

The Symptoms

We also need to take a look at some of the symptoms that are likely to show up when we are suffering from this kind of disorder. Since this condition is able to cause a lot of potential complications, it is important for us to know what some of the most common symptoms of the process are. In addition to the heartburn that we have talked about, some of the other symptoms will include:

1. Burping often. If you have burping that tastes bad, burping that you can't explain, painful burping, and more, it is a sign that there is some stomach acid in the esophagus.

2. Dark stool: The bowel movements that you are going through will say a good deal about your

health. If you are dealing with dark stools, it is a sign that something is wrong with your digestive system.

3. Dysphagia: This is where we have difficulty swallowing is going to be a sign that there is something wrong with your health, and it is best to get help from a medical doctor as soon as possible.

4. Nausea

5. Unexplained weight loss

6. A sore through that is prolonged and unexplained. It can include a sore throat that keeps coming back.

7. Tasting stomach acid on a regular basis.

8. Pain when you lay down. When you lay down, it makes it even easier for your acid in the stomach to creep into the throat, especially if your sphincter isn't really working.

9. Hiccups on a regular basis

10. Wheezing and dry cough along with hoarseness of voice.

11. Discomfort and burning pain right below the breastbone in the body, though it can potentially reach the area of the throat.

In addition, whenever there is any change in the comfort or the health that you are dealing with, it is a good idea for you to go and seek help from a medical professional. Many conditions are going to contribute to these symptoms, but keep in mind that it is possible that the acid reflux could be the culprit.

Chapter 2

HOW THE SYMPTOMS OF ACID REFLUX AND FOOD RELATE

With this in mind, it is important for us to take a look at how the foods that we eat and the symptoms of acid reflux are going to relate to one another. You will find that a combination of slow low-carbs, good fats, and lean proteins can not only be important for helping us to lose weight, but also helping us to lower the risk that we have fore GERD, and can limit the acid reflux that we are able to work with. When we feed the body the foods it needs, and we lose weight, our risks will go down.

Lowering the intake of foods that are higher in sugars, and the ones that are unhealthy and will cause issues can really impact the amount of risk that we are able to have with developing GERD. In fact, research over time has concluded that it is likely that our simple carbs (which includes sugars), could contribute more to GERD as compared to dietary fats and other options that are usually associated with this condition.

Another option that we are able to work with is our digestive enzymes and consuming some of these can help us to break down more of the proteins and fats better. This helps us to digest these foods more conveniently in the stomach. This means that when we add these to the diet, a few symptoms like gas and bloating are less likely to happen.

Alkalinity and Acidity

While we are not going to dive into this too much, we need to take a look at how acidity and alkalinity are able to work in our bodies in helping us to get things done with a healthier body. When we are dealing with acid reflux, the acid in our bodies is higher, and we are not balanced at all. But if we are able to reduce that a bit, and bring our bodies back to being slightly alkaline, then we will be able to reduce and maybe even eliminate it, and all of that can be done with some healthy life choices and good foods.

To start, when we look at the scale for pH, 0 is going to be considered acidic, and then acidic is alkaline. The pH of 7 is going to be considered to be the neutral one, which is the pH of water. These levels are going to change and vary quite a bit in our bodies, and usually, we are slightly one way or another.

Having a little bit of acidity in the body is fine. But the problem comes in when we are getting way too high on that, and we end up with a mess on our hands. Our body is not able to heal and take care of itself, and we are going to feel sick and unhealthy.

If we are able to watch some of the foods that we consume, and we take better care of our bodies, we will be able to get things back in line. Being slightly alkaline (there is no reason to go all the way over to the 0 but being slightly off the seven is a good place to be), we can help to balance the body and make it healthier.

This is why a lot of people go on a diet that is similar to the alkaline diet. This helps us to fight off some of the acids that are in the body and keeps us to the more normal and neutral manner. This kind of diet allows us to eat some good lean meats, lots of healthy fruits and vegetables and keeps some of the carbs that we eat down to a minimum. Those who follow this kind of diet are allowed to have carbs, but they must be high-quality and more, rather than the sugars and processed carbs that are found in the traditional American diet.

While many people spend a lot of time and money searching around for the right medication, and feel like they need to live in agony for the rest of their lives with this, the solution is simple. Often the foods that we eat, and the different lifestyle choices that we make like exercising and being active, are the best ways to get our bodies back in shape and prevent the acid. It is such a simple thing, but choosing wholesome and healthy foods can ensure that we are going to see the results that we want, without having to worry about expensive medications or dealing with the pain for the rest of our lives.

As we go through this guidebook, we will show you a bunch of healthy and delicious options that you can have for any meal of the day. This is not a big diet that is going to uproot your life, taste horrible, and be too hard to work with. Once you have had a chance to get over some of the sugar cravings and learn some new recipes and cooking styles, you will find that this is one of the easiest and most effective ways to deal with your acid reflux.

You will often find that the best way to deal with your acid reflux is to make sure that you are eating the right foods along the way. There are a lot of foods that are found in the American diet that may taste amazing, but they are not very good for us to use on a frequent basis. And many times, these are the foods that are causing our reflux to get as bad as it is. It is much better for us to learn more about eating right, and how this is going to make a world of difference in order to help us to get rid of our acid reflux in the process.

The foods that we eat are meant to make sure that we are healthy and strong along the way. They will be the tools that we utilize to ensure that we get things in line and that our bodies get the nutrients that we need. When we eat a lot of fast foods and other things that are full of sugars and bad carbs and not that good for us, hen we are going to end up with a big mess in our bodies. We may be filling our stomachs, but we are not going to provide our bodies with healthy nutrients and more that they really need, and this can cause trouble.

Our bodies need lots of good nutrition to help us stay healthy. Even when we just sit around and do hardly anything during the day, it takes a good deal of energy to keep our heats moving, to help us to breathe in and out to help us think, and so much more. And we are not getting the nutrients that we need from our foods when we eat sugars and other bad things as well.

Sure, they may taste good. And often we have cravings for these and hope that we can eat them more. But falling into this trap, as well as eating portions that are too big for us to handle, is going to be a downfall to our health. Both of these situations are going to cause us to deal with horrible acid reflux that we just won't be able to get rid of along the way, at least until we are able to change up some of our dietary habits as well.

This is why we need to make some big changes in the way that we eat if we want to be able to see some good results in our health. When we feed our bodies the healthy foods that it needs, ones that are full of lots of good vitamins and minerals and low in all of the bad stuff, we can help the body to function well. when we are dealing with acid reflux, we can see what is happening with the body and how all of those bad foods are not the best choices for us to make. We see what happens when we do not take good care of our bodies, and this can be a dangerous thing to deal with as well.

On the other hand, filling our bodies full of all the good stuff can make a difference. We provide the body with all of the tools and nutrients that it needs, and this helps it to function in the proper manner that we want. This is a great way to help us get rid of the acid reflux because the body is able to handle things on its own and will see some good results.

We will take some time to look at the different types of foods that you should enjoy when you are on this kind of diet plan, the acid reflux diet. But basically, you want to make sure that you are going with foods that are healthy and wholesome for the body. Going with low carb foods and only focusing on ones that have the healthy carbs you need, lots of lean meats and even fish, and lots of fruits and vegetables are the way to go to ensure that you are feeding your body all of the great nutrients that it needs to do so well.

In addition to taking care of the food that your body is eating and ensuring that you are giving it the very best, you want to double-check that you are taking care of other parts of your health as well. Doing some workouts and being active on a regular basis, socializing with those around you, and spending time doing things that you love, which can really reduce the levels of stress that you may be dealing with, can all be good options to help you get your acid reflux levels down while improving the overall standard of your health. Taking care of yourself is something that takes time and requires a lot of different parts coming together with one another, but when you are able to do this, it makes a world of difference in how well you feel.

The foods that you eat will have a big impact on your overall health and how good you are going to feel. If you are dealing with acid reflux and all of the bad things that come with it, you are likely to find that making some changes to your diet and the foods that you eat can make a world of difference in your health and how well you are going to feel in the process. When you are ready to get started with the acid reflux diet, make sure to really focus on some of the foods you eat, as well as the portions, and it will not take too long before you start to see some big improvements along the way.

Chapter 3

THE BATTLE OF THE PH

Now it is time for us to dive a bit more into the idea of pH and what this all entails. Think back to sitting in science class and listening to your teacher talks about things like pH levels and alkaline levels. You learned that one end of the scale was considered the bases, and then the other side was acidic, and you probably took some time to do experiments to help you figure this out as well.

The human body can also be found on this scale of pH in several manners. Each part of your body is on the scale in a different place, and as you can imagine, the stomach is going to be more on the acidic side of the scale. But then we have the blood that is more on the alkaline side of the scale. All of the other organs and parts of the body will be all across the board.

However, one thing that can be a bit surprising when you deal with this process is that for those who struggle with acid reflux, you are dealing with a very low amount of acid in the stomach. Many people make the assumption that when you get reflux, you have too much acid in the stomach, and it will creep on through the sphincter. But in many situations, it is not true, and in fact, it is a sign that you do not have enough acid in the stomach.

Remember here that the stomach is supposed to be like a holding compartment for all of the acids that are found there. This is the location where the acid is originally created, and it is where the acid should be stored, and all of the food is broken down quite a bit before it is able to finish the journey through the digestive tract.

When we deal with the acid reflux that we are exploring here, you will find that the acid that is found and created in your stomach is going to make its way to the esophagus, resulting in a lower amount of acid in the stomach because it moved. It is no surprise here that your body is a system that is going to work with itself in a lot of different manners, and when one part of the system is no longer in balance, then the other parts are going to struggle and lose their balance as well.

Another surprising fact is that a lot of times, the foods that we eat will have a lot of effects on our body. Many of the foods found on the list of triggers are going to be the foods that will cause the body as a whole to become more acidic than before. And this is not a good thing for those dealing with acid reflux.

The goal of working with the acid reflux diet is to consume foods on a regular basis that is not going to cause your condition to become worse and to incorporate foods that will bring your body back into the pH balance that it should as you shop, cook, and eat. It can help us to look for foods that will give your body the desired effect that you would like to achieve.

There are a lot of resources that you are able to find all over the place that will list out all of the different foods and where they actually fall on the pH scale. It is good to look into some of those and then bases some of your shopping, and then the cooking you do, on the levels of pH in the foods you want to eat. This can be a safe, effective, ad easy manner to help you to cut down on the levels of acidity in the body and help you balance again.

A good place to start with this is to make a list of foods that you eat ad the way that they affect your body personally. Some people can eat foods that are higher in acidity, and it doesn't affect them as much. Each body is going to be a bit different, and learning what your body can tolerate, and what it can't, is one of the best ways to get things in order. You can always talk to your doctor about this too, and ask them about what you should choose when acid reflux is an issue.

There are many charts and graphs that you can look at to get a good outline of where to start. You can try out some of those foods and look at how you feel once they are gone and out of your diet. Then, if you want to see which ones are specifically going to cause you harm and discomfort, slowly reintroduce one or two back at a time. If one of them starts to make you get sick again and starts the acid reflux up again, then you know you have a sensitivity to that and should avoid it. If you can enjoy it for a week or two without issues, then you can keep that one on your diet and not get rid of it.

This is a slow process, and it can take months to figure out exactly which foods are fine for you and which ones are going to cause a few issues along the way. But eliminating all of them in the beginning, and slowly bringing them back in once your body settles into a new normal, is a good way to make sure that you figure out the exact foods that are good for you, and the ones that you need to watch out for.

This is why it is so important to work with your body to figure out what works for you and then opt for the foods that will help you feel your best. This could be a similar list to what you find online, but then there may be some foods on the list that you are just fine with, and other foods that you may have a sensitivity to and need to avoid. The end goal here is that you want to get rid of the symptoms of acid reflux, regardless of how well you follow a list for your own body. The lists online are a good place to start, but you may have to make some adjustments for your own self.

Remember that in addition to this, the more that you are able to learn about all of the different kinds of foods that you put into your body, and the different things that the food is going to do to your body, the better off you will be when making good decisions for your own health. Yes, this is a process that takes some time, and you will need to put in a good deal of effort in order to make it happen. But you will soon find that it is all worth it. No cost can match good health, and though this can take time and be frustrating sometimes, it is important for helping you to be in control over your own body and the health it is in at any given time.

This brings us back to some of the importance of why we want to have a balanced level of pH in our bodies. The balance between acidity and the alkalinity in the body is going to be known as pH, or the potential of hydrogen. There are a variety of factors that are going to help us determine whether our blood has too much, or too little acid, and it can include things like the overall health of our organs and how well they are able to get the carbon dioxide out of the body, and even the foods that you eat.

You will find that it is actually a pretty complex process to get your pH balances in check inside of the body, and even when you do some of the right steps and take care of your body, there are times when some stress or other environmental factors are going to throw it out. The good news, though, is that it is possible to regulate it and keep it as close to being balanced as possible, with some healthy habits.

Remember that we talked about how the level of pH that we have is going to be found on a scale that goes from 0 to 14. The lower the pH level, the more acidic something is. But the higher the level of pH, the more alkaline. And then we end up with a neutral pH, like that of water, at 7.0. the healthy range for most people will be somewhere between 6.0 and 7.5 depending on the day and how they live their lives.

According to what is found on the Merck Manuals Online Medical Library, blood that is slightly alkaline, or falls somewhere between 7.35 and 7.45 is going to be the most optimal for your body to function well. This is why this kind of diet plan is going to focus on meeting this range as much as possible. When you eat foods that are alkaline and avoid the ones that are acidic, you are able to get your own body into balance and ensure that your body and the organs are able to function well.

It is common for many people, especially those in the western world, to have an imbalance that makes them more acidic than they should be. When this happens, thanks to the unhealthy diet that they deal with, it is going to lead to a lot of health ailments. Not only are they going to deal with things like acid reflux and GERD< they could deal with other issues like frail bones, complications with diabetes, and even heart disease.

If this is something that happens on a regular basis, we could end up with some complications of the lungs and kidneys. Respiratory or metabolic acidosis is going to happen when we have an excess amount of acid in the blood for a long period of time. When we see the metabolic acidosis, this means that we are going to have a metabolism that is abnormal from the buildup of ketones in the blood. This can occur in things like the overuse of aspirin or alcohol, or diabetes that is not controlled, and all result in the kidneys not being able to do their jobs in the proper manner.

When we take a look at the respiratory acidosis, you find that your lungs struggle to get rid of the carbon dioxide found in the well, which can result in a number of problems like pneumonia and asthma. Symptoms could include a lot of things like confusion, weakness, breathing complications, fatigue, and committing to naming a few of them. And if you do not follow some of the guidance in this guidebook and make some quick changes in your lifestyle and your health, then this acidosis can lead to the constriction of the blood vessels, lung collapse, and kidney failure.

Now, we want to make sure that when we make some changes in the body, we are doing so in a healthy and balanced way. This diet is not going to tell you to never have another acidic food again. It is just going to focus on going with foods that are healthier and can give you the best balance possible.

The reason that we bring this up is that there is a problem known as alkalosis. This is going to be the opposite problem that we would see with acidosis, and it happens when there is too much bicarbonate in the blood, which means that the body is too alkaline. When you overuse diuretics, and you work with hyperventilating too much, then you will find that there is too much carbon dioxide that shows up in the blood.

When you are dealing with this kind of alkalosis, it can also be respiratory or metabolic as well. and it is going to have a few symptoms that include irritability, cramps, and muscular twitching. The best way to help with this is to replace your fluids so that you can get back to the right acid balance, or if you are dealing with the issue of respiratory alkalosis, you will work on slowing down your rate of breathing a little bit.

The main goal here is to make sure that you are able to maintain your levels of pH, not let them get too far one way or the other. And one of the best ways to help with this is to make sure that you eat the right foods that can maintain this balance. There are a number of foods that are considered really acidic to deal with and should be kept to a minimum as much as possible. These are going to include:

1. Cheese
2. Beef
3. Walnuts
4. Chocolate
5. Blackberries
6. Prunes

You can also go through and make some changes to what you are eating to include foods that are seen as more alkaline in nature. These can help you to reduce the amount of acid that is found in the body and will keep you healthier and happier in the long run. Some of the options that you can go with include olive oil, spinach, asparagus, and watermelon, to name a few.

To make sure that you are able to maintain your pH balance as much as possible, go with vegetables, grains, and fruits that are going to be seen as middle acidic or alkaline, and then only go with the higher acidic foods when you know your pH level is starting to get too far over to the alkaline side of things. You can also hydrate with a lot of water on a daily basis, limit the amount of alcohol that you consume, and always take your medication in the right manner so that you can prevent your pH levels from getting too high.

As we can see, there are a lot of benefits that come with keeping our pH levels in check and making sure that we are not going too much over or too much under on the pH level at all. Making sure that our bodies are not too acidic is one of the best ways to help maintain our health and make sure that we are not going to suffer from things like acid reflux or any of the other conditions that are related to this. We will look at some of the recipes that you are able to focus on later to help you to get your pH levels back in check and to help you to get things done in no time as well. The acid reflux diet is one of the best ways to improve your health and to get you back on track for a healthier lifestyle as well.

Chapter 4

SIMPLE TREATMENT OPTIONS

In this chapter, we are going to take a look at some of the simple treatment options that we are able to use when it comes to working with the acid reflux we feel. Whether we just deal with it on occasion or it is something that we experience a few times a week on a regular basis, acid reflux is painful and not much fun in the process.

The good news is that there are a ton of different treatment options that we are able to work with depending on what we hope to achieve with this, and how often and severe the acid reflux is all about. Let's dive into this and learn more about acid reflux and some of the different treatments that you can use to get yours under control.

Medications

One of the first places people go when they want to deal with their acid reflux is straight to the doctor to get some medication. Sure the acid and all of the symptoms that come with it are painful and not fun, and we worry about what it is doing to the esophagus and other parts of the body at the same time. Many people worry that this is going to get out of hand, and they worry about their health, so they run to get help from medication.

Now, not all medication is a bad thing. It can really provide the relief that you are looking for if you use it in the proper manner. And if you have tried a lot of other natural remedies and have worked really hard on your diet and the acid is just not getting better, then medication may be the best option for you.

There are two main types of medications that a patient is able to utilize to help them deal with their acid reflux. First are the antacids. These are things like Tums, though there are stronger options that the doctor can prescribe, which will act in a way to neutralize the acids in the stomach. And the acids in the stomach are neutralized; it means that acid reflux can go away, and it can provide some quick relief. If you are someone who only gets acid reflux on occasion, then these are probably going to be a quick way for you to make it go away without needing anything too serious.

It is also possible to work with a medication that is known as H-2 receptor blockers. These are not going to be able to act in a manner that is as quick as the antacids, but they are going to be able to provide us with relief that is a lot longer, and they could decrease the amount of acid that is produced in the stomach for 12 hours or more, which can be better for those who suffer from acid reflux on a regular basis.

Procedures

In some situations, it is possible that you will need to take the work of your acid reflux to the next level, and you may need to get some kind of procedure done in order to deal with it. This can often be done to help with the sphincter if it is really weak, and none of the other options that are tried have actually worked.

The first procedure that we are able to take a look at here is the Linx surgery. This is where the surgeon is going to wrap a ring of tiny beads around the LES. This ring is going to be strong enough that it can keep the opening closed to some of the acids that are trying to keep up, but loose enough that the food you eat is still able to come down through it. It is a great way to ensure that you are not going to have to worry about the weak sphincter any more.

Then there is a procedure that is known as the Nissen fundoplication. This is where we take the upper part of the stomach, and then we wrap it around the lower part of the esophageal sphincter. This is going to work because it prevents the reflux from getting back into the esophagus when it wants.

These procedures are going to carry some risks, and it is not common for people to go through these to deal with their acid reflux unless it is really severe, and none of the other options are going to cut it. It is much better for us to go through and monitor our diet, look at some of the natural remedies, and even try some medications first because those will usually be perfect, and a lot safer, ways to help us deal with our conditions instead of surgery.

Nutrition

While all of the other options are going to be great for helping you to deal with your acid reflux, if you are dealing with this condition on a regular basis, then it is time to make some changes, and we need to make them right now. It is likely that our environment, along with the foods that we are consuming, are some of the major culprits when it comes to dealing with this issue, and that is why we need to always make sure that when acid reflux is an issue, that we worry about the foods that we take in.

Eating the right foods, and avoiding the foods that are bad for us, are the best ways to get started with this. First, we need to provide our bodies with lots of healthy and wholesome foods. We will look at a more extensive list for this in a moment, but basically, the diet that you want to consume when avoiding your acid reflux and all of the negative symptoms that come with that include egg whites and lean meats, non-citrus fruits, oatmeal, ginger, and other herbs, and even vegetables.

But the foods that you avoid are going to be important as well. if you eat a lot of the foods that are on the not allowed list, then it is more likely that your reflux is going to at up a bit more again, and this can cause more damage to the body. Some of the things that we want to be careful about when we are dealing with acid and want to get rid of it include mint, caffeine, garlic, spicy foods and onion, chocolates, tomatoes, citrus fruits, and any foods that are higher in fat content. Eating too much of these will cause the body to become more acidic overall.

When you are able to shift your ideas on how to eat, and start to focus on eating some of the good things that can fuel your body and will provide you with some of the nutrients and minerals that you need to do well in life, you will be able to fight off some of the acid and the symptoms that come with acid along the way. It is not always easy to work with, and sometimes you will want to give in (and if you do this occasionally and not all of the time, that is fine), but overall, it can help lead you to much better health.

Natural Remedies

In addition to some of the medications and other options that we discussed in the last part, there are a few options that we can use that are considered more natural remedies. These can work really well in helping keep the body in line and balanced, and sometimes work better than the medications and other options above, without all of the negative side effects that go along with it. Some of the more natural options and remedies that you can use for GERD and acid reflux will include:

1. Organic Honey, Indian Gooseberry, and Fresh Basil

Some of the remedies that we are able to talk about are going to include natural and holistic foods, along with some herbal therapies. One of these is organic honey that is unrefined. This is cheap, simple, and available to try out with reducing the burning that happens with the reflux. The honey is a natural way to help cut down on the pH and taking even just a bit at bedtime could be a great way to calm down the issues when you go to bed.

Fresh basil is a good option here. This is going to be a remedy that can relieve acid reflux. Sometimes just chewing on the fresh basil leaves will be enough, but there is also some basil tea in health food stores that can work well to help calm the system and is often preferable to eating it raw. Along with this, Indian gooseberry is a good herb to use here that will help with protecting the digestive tract and all that is found in it against stomach acid.

2. Slippery Elm, Bromelain, and Licorice Root

Another option is the licorice root, which is going to be a good soothing agent since it is able to build up some protective layers in the esophagus, and you can get it as a tea as well. it is recommended that you watch out a bit for your blood pressure with this one, though, because some people have noted that it will go up. Deglycyrrhized licorice is another good option because it is going to come in a tablet and is soothing and calming.

Next on the list is Bromelain. This is one of the enzymes in a pineapple, so you can take just the enzyme or eat some pineapple after your meals to help digest your food. This particular enzyme is going to help move the food faster, so it doesn't irritate your stomach.

We can also work with something known as slippery elm. This is a good one to coat the stomach, similar to what gooseberry can do. It often works with the gooseberry to keep the stomach healthy and strong along the way.

3. Baking Soda, Apple Cider Vinegar, and Cayenne Pepper

Cayenne pepper and apple cider vinegar. When we hear both of these, we assume it is a misprint and that neither of these will work. When it comes to cayenne pepper, we know that it is a pepper that is hot and burning, and we assume that it is going to make the situation worse. But for some people, it can be an effective way to heal inflammation and the ulcers that come with it. If you add a bit of apple cider vinegar to water as well, you can help with this because it makes digestion go more smoothly overall.

Some people save the apple cider vinegar for when the acid reflux is really bad. But other times, just having it on a regular basis may be the solution you need. Having about an ounce before or after your meals, especially in those who frequently have to deal with heartburn, can help make the situation go away.

If you are in a pinch and need to deal with acid reflux, then some baking soda is going to be the best option. This is an antacid though, so if you have a low stomach production of this acid, it is sometimes better to go with something like the apple cider vinegar instead. It can work on occasion, but it isn't something that we should do all of the time.

4. Eat Slowly and Keep the Meals Small

A big thing that anyone can do, whether they are dealing with heartburn or not, is to slow down and chew their food. If you eat the food slowly, and you take the time to chew it up, you will be able to digest the part of it with enzymes in your mouth. That way, when it does go down, it will have an easier time moving through the stomach and getting digested and can help keep the heartburn and the acid away from you.

Another thing along these lines to remember is that you should avoid large, fatty, and greasy meals. Slow down when eating healthy and wholesome foods, eat smaller meals, eat slower, and you will find that it is a lot easier to handle the acid and keep it away.

5. Digestive Enzymes and Probiotics

Both of these are going to be important to make sure that the digestion is going to work well or us. We need to make sure that all of the bacteria that is supposed to be in our guts, helping us to digest our food and take care of things, will work up to code, or it can cause a lot of issues for us.

When these bacteria are not flourishing (and these are the good kinds that are supposed to be there and help us), then our digestion is going to fail, we will feel bad, and often acid reflux is going to be one of the issues that we need to deal with in the process. Adding in a probiotic and some digestive enzymes can be the trick that we need to make these flourish again and get things back on track.

6. Essential Oils

Some people like to work with essential oils to help them deal with some of the issues of acid reflux. There are a few different options that are said to help with these. DoTerra is a good option to use because they see a capsule or oils that you can use to fight off the reflux, and it includes things like essential oils, coriander, anise, caraway fennel, tarragon, pepper, and ginger.

All of those ingredients have been used on their own to help out with these intestinal problems. But when you are able to combine them with one another, it could be the best way to soothe heartburn and calm down the stomach. And since there are no side effects that come from using this option, you can bet it is one of the best to help you handle your acid reflux as well.

As we can see, there are a number of different options that you are able to choose when it comes to handling your acid reflux and making sure that you get it under control. Each one can be effective, but along with the foods that you are allowed to eat and the ones that you should avoid, each person is going to react to the methods in different ways.

It is best if you are able to take some time to learn how to work with these and learn which one is the best for your needs. Some people find that just taking a peppermint after a meal is effective, and others may try the natural remedies and find that they are not strong enough, so they will switch over to some medications. Finding the solution that works the best for you is the most important part here, and when you are able to do that, you will find that it is easier for you to get relief from acid reflux.

Chapter 5

FOOD LISTS

Now that we have had some fun learning more about the issues with acid reflux and what can cause it, and we even have a good idea on some of the remedies that we can use in order to get the acid reflux under control for some of our own needs, it is time to look at the foods we eat. One of the easiest and most effective ways to deal with our acid reflux before it is able to take over our lives and ruin our health is to eat the right kinds of foods. And this is exactly what we are going to talk about in this guidebook to help us get started.

The Foods to Avoid

First on the list is some of the foods that you are not allowed to eat. Remember that if you want, you can do the elimination diet and take some of them out for a bit, adding them back in later to see if they actually cause any issues. But to start this diet out, and to help reduce the amount of inflammation that we are dealing with, we need to avoid these foods as much as possible. The foods below are going to be known to make GERD worse, and they are more acidic than others. Try to limit or reduce their intake as much as you can:

1. Foods that are high in oils and fats. These foods can cause the sphincter in the stomach to relax a bit, and that will make the acid reflux worse.

2. Meats that are fatty. These are known to be highly acidic because they have higher amounts of cholesterols and fatty acids in them.

3. Foods that are going to be the sources of saturated fats in our diet. These can include options like whole milk and full-fat cheese.

4. Lots of salt. Having a bit of sodium in your diet is not a bad thing. But if you are going way over the limits that are given to the standard American diet, and most Americans are, then it is best to reduce this as much as possible.

5. Mint

6. Chocolate

7. Sodas and other carbonated beverages

8. Caffeine

9. Drinks that are known to be more acidic such as orange juice and coffee.

10. Foods that are more acidic such as tomato sauce.

It is important that if you would like to reduce the amount of acid reflux that you are dealing, and you want to make sure that you keep your health conditions from this issue down to a minimum, that you are able to go through and avoid the foods that are above as much as possible. Having them on occasion is not always bad, and sometimes they can be a nice treat. But if they consist of most of your diet and most of the foods that you consume, then that is not a good thing and can cause a lot of harm to your body as well.

The Foods to Enjoy

Now that we have been able to go through a list of foods that you need to avoid when you are on this diet in order to maintain your health, and now that you may be feeling that a lot of your favorite food choices are gone, it is time for us to take a look at some of the great food choices that are allowed on this diet plan. These are the foods that are known to be more alkaline, and that will result in them helping you avoid the risk of having GERD at all. You are more than welcome to consume these in abundance and can have as much as you would like. Some of the foods that fit in with this list include:

1. Carbs that are present in some of the different veggies and fruits that are considered low in acid. Certain whole grains are fine as well.

2. Proteins that come from lean sources like lean poultry without the skin, lentils, trout, salmon, and beans. We want to make sure that the protein source we use is going to be low in cholesterol levels.

3. Foods that have a higher content of Vitamin C in them. This would include the fruits that are low in acid and vegetables.

4. Green vegetables like kale, broccoli, Brussels sprouts, asparagus, and spinach to help fill us up and give us a lot of the nutrients that we are looking for.

5. Foods that are higher in fiber. We want to focus on those that are high in soluble fiber because this

kind is going to help us lower the risk of GERD as well.

6. Fruits that are high in fiber and have a lot of magnesium and potassium. This would include options like berries, pears, peaches, bananas, avocados, melons, and apples.

7. Eggs. It doesn't matter what their cholesterol levels are. These are still allowed on the diet.

8. Foods that increase the acidity of the body should not be on your diet plan.

9. Eat foods that are considered to be more alkaline in nature.

10. Eat lots of fruits and veggies, and things like bananas, spinach, and broccoli are great on this kind of plan.

As we can see, there are still a lot of great foods that we are able to consume and enjoy when we are on this kind of diet plan. Using it will ensure that we have a chance to really enjoy the meals we eat and fill up our bodies with things that are healthy and good for us, rather than all of the bad substances that are just causing us pain and misery in the process.

One thing that we have to remember here is that the foods on the first list are not completely off bounds all of the time. It is fine to splurge on occasion, and maybe have a soda or some chocolate on occasion. This is not to say that you should never have them. But if you are suffering from acid reflux, then there is a problem, and you should make sure to eliminate these as much as possible along the way. Having them as a treat on occasion can make it more fun and probably won't harm you too much unless you are really sensitive, but you should not get into the habit of having these each day with all of your meals, or the acid reflux will come back.

Chapter 6

THE ONE-WEEK MEAL PLAN

As we mentioned, one of the best ways that we can make sure we take care of ourselves and reduce the amount of acid reflux that we are dealing with on a regular basis is to watch the foods that we eat. The things that we put into our bodies are really important, and it is important that we take care of them all the time. The foods we eat are not always the best, and while this doesn't mean we have to give up some of the good stuff all of the time, it does mean that we need to take more precautions to take care of ourselves and pay attention.

Eating the traditional American diet isn't good for anyone. It may taste great, and it may be easy and make us feel good for the short time that we do it. But the acid reflux, along with the obesity and other health conditions that you are most likely suffering from, are signs that this form of nutrition is not that good for us. That is why the major focus that shows up when people are dealing with acid reflux that won't go away is that they need to learn how to change their diets.

Yes, you will need to give up some of your old favorite foods and start focusing on things that are a lot healthier and good for you. The sugar cravings and the need for caffeine may be strong as well. but you will find that when you switch over and find some good and tasty meals and recipes to help you do this, things are going to get a whole lot easier in the long run.

That is why the rest of this guidebook is going to take some time to look at the different steps you can take to make sure your diet and nutrition are on par for your health and for stopping acid reflux. Below, we are going to show you a great meal plan that you are able to follow, one that will make it easier for you to get in good health, eliminate some of the bad foods for you, and focus on the good ones that can help keep your acid reflux in check, and improve so many other aspects of your health at the same time.

With that in mind, here is the meal plan that you can follow when you are ready to follow the acid reflux diet, and you are ready to get your health back on track.

Day 1:

Breakfast: Quinoa Porridge

Lunch: Potato Medley Soup

Dinner: Baked Herb Tilapia

Day 2:

Breakfast: Banana Bread

Lunch: Crab Cakes

Dinner: Simple Vegetable Broth

Day 3:

Breakfast: Vegetable Tacos

Lunch: Halibut and Veggie Packets

Dinner: Roast Beef

Day 4:

Breakfast: Sweet Potato Tarts

Lunch: Coconut Panko Shrimp

Dinner: Broccoli and Cheese Baked Potato

Day 5:

Breakfast: English Muffins

Lunch: Chicken Noodle Soup

Dinner: Salmon and Lentils

Day 6:

Breakfast: Fruit and Yogurt Parfait

Lunch: Italian Vegetable Soup

Dinner: Inside-Out Cabbage Rolls

Day 7:

Breakfast: Chia Quinoa

Lunch: Easy Tuna Melt

Dinner: Lamb Chops

CHAPTER 7: EASY BREAKFAST RECIPES

MORNING PORRIDGE

What's Inside:

- Salt
- Vanilla (.5 tsp.)
- Splenda (3 Tbsp.)
- Almond milk, low-fat (1.5 c.)
- Quinoa (.75 c)

How to Make This:

1. Take out a cooking pot and add in the milk. Let the milk reach a boil and then whisk in the quinoa.

2. Stir and cook this whole mixture in the milk until it becomes creamy and smooth.

3. Add in Splenda, vanilla, and salt to the mixture, stir it around again, and then serve warm.

BANANA BREAD

What's Inside:

- Bananas, peeled (3)
- Almond butter, melted (.33 c.)
- Baking soda (1 tsp.)
- Coconut flour (1.5 c.)
- Splenda (.75 c.)
- Salt
- Vanilla (1 tsp.)

How to Make This:

1. Turn on the oven and let it have time to heat up to 350 degrees. While the oven is getting nice and hot, take out a bread pan and use some almond butter to grease it all up.

2. Bring out a glass bowl at this time and mash up the bananas inside of it. Whisk in the rest of the almond butter that you melted.

3. Mix the salt and the baking soda inside of another bowl. When these are combined well, add in the vanilla, Splenda, and the egg that is whisked. Stir in the flour and get it all to mix well.

4. Add the bananas here to it all before transferring to the prepared pan that you got to earlier. Add to the over.

5. When 50 minutes or so are done, you can take this out of the oven. Allow it time to cool down before slicing into it and serving.

FRENCH TOAST

What's Inside:

- Butter (1 tsp.)
- Sandwich bread without gluten (4 slices)
- Salt
- Nutmeg (.5 tsp.)
- Stevia (1 packet)
- Orange zest, grated (1 tsp.)
- Vanilla (.5 tsp.)
- Beaten eggs (2)
- Nonfat milk (1.5 c.)

How to Make This:

1. To start, take out a bowl and whisk together the salt, nutmeg, stevia, orange zest, vanilla, eggs, and milk.

2. Pour all of these mixed ingredients into a shallow dish. Add in the bread and soak it into this for a few minutes, making sure to flip around to coat on all sides.

3. Take out a skillet and heat it up with a bit of butter on top. When the butter is melted, add on the bread to bake.

4. After two or three minutes on each side, the custard on the bread should set and brown. You can then

serve this with some of your favorite berries or other toppings.

BANANA PANCAKES

What's Inside:

- Butter (1 tsp.)
- Beaten eggs (2)
- Peeled banana ripe (1)

How to Make This:

1. To start this recipe, take out a small bowl. Place a banana inside and then mash it all up.

2. When the banana is all done being mashed up, add in the eggs and whisk them up to combine.

3. Take out a skillet and heat it up. Add on the butter and give it some time to melt.

4. When the skillet is all ready, scoop the banana mixture and place it on the skillet. It should make four pancakes.

5. Cook these for a minute on each side and then serve warm.

SWEET POTATO HASH

What's Inside:

- Salt (.5 tsp.)
- Dried thyme (.5 tsp.)
- Cubed sweet potatoes (1)
- Olive oil (1 Tbsp.)

How to Make This:

1. Take out a skillet and hit it up on a medium-high heat setting. Add in the oil and let it heat up until it starts to shimmer.

2. Add in the thyme, salt, and sweet potatoes. Cook these until the potatoes are starting to brown a bit.

3. After four minutes have passed, you can lower the heat a little bit. Continue to cook for a bit longer, until your sweet potatoes are browned.

4. This takes another 15 minutes to complete. When it is done, you can serve warm.

APRICOT OATS

What's Inside:

- Coconut, dried (.33 c.)
- Dried apricots, chopped (.5 c.)
- Rolled oats (2 c.)
- Pitted dates (.25 c.)
- Ground ginger (1 tsp.)
- Dried figs (.33 c.)
- Egg whites (5)

How to Make This:

1. When you are ready to start this recipe, turn on the oven and set it to 350 degrees. Take out the baking sheet that you want to use and add on some parchment paper.

2. Take out a bowl and mix all of your ingredients together until well combined, leaving the whites of the eggs out.

3. When the other ingredients are mixed well, you can stir in the eggs and mix again.

4. Spread the whole mixture onto the baking tray and add it into your oven.

5. After 40 minutes of baking, take a look and see if the oats are all done, if they are, bring them out of the oven and give time to cool.

6. When it is time to serve, slice this up, and enjoy it.

VEGGIE TACOS

What's Inside:

- Olive oil (1 Tbsp.)
- Salt
- Sliced and peeled carrot (1)
- Diced sweet potato (1)
- Coriander, ground (.5 tsp.)
- Lime zest (.5 tsp.)
- Cumin, ground (1 tsp.)
- Corn tortillas (120
- Black beans in a can and mashed (1 c.)
- Olive oil (1 Tbsp.)

How to Make This:

1. To start this recipe, turn on the oven and allow it some time to heat up to 350 degrees. Take out a cookie sheet while that heats up and line with some baking paper.

2. In the meantime, mix the sweet potatoes and carrots with some oil, lime zest, cumin, coriander, and salt in a smaller bowl.

3. Move this whole mixture over to that prepared cookie sheet and then add it all to the oven to roast.

4. After 15 minutes or so, the vegetables should be done. Take them out of the oven and provide them with time to cool down.

5. Take the tortillas out and spread the beans on top of it. Top it all with some vegetables before serving.

EASY SMOOTHIES

What's Inside:

- Grated ginger, peeled (.5 tsp.)
- Milk, low fat (1.5 c.)
- Ice (1 c.)
- Fat-free yogurt without flavor (1 c.)
- Bananas (2)
- Honey (1 Tbsp.)

How to Make This:

1. Take out your food processor and get it all set up in order to use it. Peel the banana and then chop it inside of the prepared food processor.

2. Add in the milk yogurt, ice, and ginger to the food processor and blend this until the consistency is nice and smooth.

3. Add in the honey as the last thing here and then blend for a few more seconds as well.

4. Pour into a few glasses and then serve when ready.

MANGO SMOOTHIE

What's Inside:

- Chopped mango (1)
- Ice cubes
- Pink small fruit in segments (1)
- Chopped banana peeled (1)
- Yogurt, natural and free of fat (2 c.)

How to Make This:

1. Take out your blender and get it all set up to start this recipe.

2. When the blender is ready, take out the yogurt, ice cubes, banana, pink fruit, and mango.

3. Blend these all together inside of your blender until they reach the consistency that you would like. Pour into your favorite glass and serve.

SWEET POTATO TARTS

What's Inside:

- Maple syrup (1 Tbsp.)
- Filtered water (4 quarts)
- Cookies, ginger snap (4 oz.) salt
- Vanilla (2 tsp>0
- Milk (.75 c)
- Sweet potatoes (20 oz.)
- Eggs, large (2)

How to Make This:

1. To get this recipe started, turn on the oven and let it have time to heat up to 325 degrees.

2. While that is heating up, we can take out a big pot and place some water inside. Put it on the stove and let it heat up to high.

3. Add in the sweet potatoes. When you see that the water is boiling, reduce the heat a bit and let it go at a simmer.

4. The sweet potatoes need to cook until they are soft and can be mashed up or have a knife slip through the middle. This can take about 35 minutes to accomplish.

5. When this is done, take the sweet potatoes out of the pot and then add them to a plate that has been

lined with paper towels. Give them some time to cool.

6. During this time, bring out the food processor and add your ginger snaps inside with a steel blade to help crumble these up into medium-sized crumbs.

7. Pulse the processor while you drizzle in some of the maple syrup.

8. When this is done, take out some foil papers to help you to line up your muffin tins along the way.

9. Then it is time to distribute, as evenly as possible, the ginger snaps cookie mixture in foil into the muffin cups. Take the time to pat down gently.

10. Add these into the oven and allow them to cook for a bit. After about 10 minutes, take this muffin tin out of the oven.

11. Mash the prepared sweet potatoes until they are smooth. Then bring out a bowl and add these along with the egg yolks, milk, Splenda, vanilla, and salt in one bowl.

12. In a separate bowl, we want to whisk the egg whites until they have formed into some stiff peaks.

13. Fold the eggs into the sweet potato mixture before scooping this batter into your prepared muffin cups. Add the whole thing back into the oven.

14. After 40 minutes or so, the mixture should be done. Take it out of the oven and give it some time to cool down. Then chill and serve.

SWEET POTATO TOAST

What's Inside:

- Kiwis, peeled (2)
- Sweet potato, peeled (1)
- Honey, organic (.5 tsp.)
- Almond butter (3 Tbsp.)
- Ginger, ground (.25 tsp.)

How to Make This:

1. To start this recipe, take the sweet potato and slice it into some long slices going lengthways.

2. Take out a bowl and stir in the ginger, almond butter, and honey until they are well combined together.

3. Turn on your toaster to the high setting and toast the sliced sweet potatoes until they are soft and cooked all the way. It is possible that you will need to do a few rounds of toasting in order to get this done.

4. When the sweet potato is done, you can spread one side of all your slices with that premade honey mixture and then top with the kiwis before serving.

MORNING CHICKEN

What's Inside:

- Olive oil (2 tsp.)
- Salt
- Fennel seed, ground (.5 tsp)
- Turmeric, ground (1 tsp.)
- Chicken breasts, skinless (4)

How to Make This:

1. Turn on the oven and give it some time to heat up to 375 degrees. While the oven is warming up, take out a cookie sheet and line with some baking paper.

2. Then bring out a bowl and mix together your fennel, turmeric, salt, and oil until they are well combined here.

3. Add the chicken breasts to your prepared cookie sheets and then brush that oil mixture you just made all over it.

4. Move the whole thing to the oven and let it bake. After 20 minutes, check the internal temperature to see if the chicken is done.

5. Take this out of the oven and allow it some time to cool down before slicing and serving.

ENGLISH MUFFINS

What's Inside:

- Almond butter, soft (3 Tbsp.)
- Instant yeast (2 tsp.)
- Almond milk (1.75 c.)
- Semolina (2 Tbsp.)
- Splenda (2 Tbsp.)
- Egg white, lightly beaten (1)
- Salt
- Coconut flour (4.5 c.)

How to Make This:

1. Take out a bowl, and except for the semolina, mix all of the ingredients for the muffins together. Bring out an electric mixer and blend these ingredients to make your dough.

2. Set the dough aside with a towel on top and let it rest for a few hours.

3. After two hours have passed, take out two muffin tins and grease them up with some cooking oil. Sprinkle some of the semolina into each cup.

4. Brin gout the dough and knead it before dividing it into 16 pieces that are as even as possible. Roll each of these 16 pieces into a small ball and add to the muffin tray.

5. Cover the muffin trays up and allow this to rest for a bit. During that 20 minutes, turn on the oven and let it heat up to 350 degrees.

6. When the oven is ready and the time is up, add the muffin tins into the oven and let them bake.

7. After 15 minutes, the muffins should be golden. Take them out and allow some time to cool before enjoying.

CORN PORRIDGE

What's Inside:

- Raisins (3 Tbsp.)
- Maple syrup (1 Tbsp.)
- Salt
- Water (2.25 c.)
- Cornmeal (.75 c.)

How to Make This:

1. Take out a bowl and add in .75 cups of water with the cornmeal. Whisk these together and set aside.

2. Take out a small pot and add in the rest o the water, along with a bit of salt. Bring the water to a boil there.

3. Whisk in the slurry of cornmeal that you made. You want to allow this to cook until the mixture is thick, which can take about 10 minutes or so.

4. When that time is up, stir in the raisins and maple syrup before serving warm.

CHIA QUINOA

What's Inside:

- Vanilla (.5 tsp.)
- Shredded coconut (1 tsp.)
- Coconut syrup (1 Tbsp.)
- Chia seeds (4 tsp.)
- Water (1 c)
- Quinoa (1 c.)
- Coconut milk (1 c.)

How to Make This:

1. To start this recipe, bring out a pan and pour your coconut milk inside. Add in the quinoa and then close the lid while placing onto the stove and turning the heat up.

2. This will allow the quinoa to cook. After about 15 minutes, the quinoa should be done. When it is done, take it from the heat and give it time to chill all the way through.

3. While the quinoa is cooking, mix together the chia seeds, water, and almond milk.

4. When the quinoa is done cooling down, add in the coconut syrup and the vanilla extract. Stir things around before adding in the chia seeds.

5. Move to the serving bowls that you want to use, decorate with a bit of the shredded coconut that

you have prepared in each bowl, and then serve this while warm.

APPLE PARFAIT

What's Inside:

- Hemp seeds (1 Tbsp)
- Chopped apples (2)
- Vanilla (.25 tsp.)
- Coconut milk (2 oz.)
- Soaked cashews (2 oz.)

How to Make This:

1. Bring out your blender and get it all set up for this one. Place the hemp seeds, vanilla, coconut milk, and cashews inside.

2. Blend this whole mixture until it is smooth and creamy.

3. After you are done with this part, add a bit of this into one of your bowls or glasses of choosing. Then add in a layer of the chopped apples on top of this.

4. You can repeat these layers back and forth until you have used up all of the ingredients. Then serve as it or let cool down first.

SCRAMBLED EGGS

What's Inside:

- Salt
- Olive oil (1 tsp.)
- Almond milk (3 tsp.)
- Rye bread without gluten (4 slices)
- Watercress (2 oz.)
- Whisked eggs (4)

How to Make This:

1. To start with this recipe, mix together the almond milk and the eggs in a bowl. Add in some salt and then stir the ingredients together slowly.

2. Take out a frying pan and add in some olive oil before preheating this. When the oil is hot, add in the mixture of whisked eggs to the pan and allow it to cook for a minute on the stove.

3. After this, we want to scramble the eggs well before cooking a few seconds more to finish this up.

4. Scramble the eggs one more time here, add the lid on top, and cook a bit longer. This will take about two more minutes to finish.

5. After we cook the scrambled eggs, we can transfer them to be on top of the rye bread and add the watercress to the top. Serve the scrambled eggs and bread when ready.

CHERRY ALMOND BAKE

What's Inside:

- Cooked quinoa (1 c.)

- Pitted cherries (1.5 c.)

- Raw almonds (.25 c.)

- Himalayan salt (.25 tsp.)

- Almond extract (.25 tsp.)
  vanilla (.75 tsp.)

- Almond meal (.33 c.)

- Pitted dates (.25 c.)

- Almond milk (3 Tbsp.)

How to Make This:

1. Turn on the oven and give it time to heat up to 350 degrees. While the oven is heating up, line a small baking dish with some parchment paper.

2. In the meantime, you can take out a food processor and combine half the cherries and half the almonds inside along with the salt, almond extract, vanilla, almond meal, dates, and almond milk.

3. Add this mixture, after you have pulsed it, into a big bowl and add in the quinoa. Pour into the baking dish that you prepared and add the rest of the almonds and cherries on top.

4. Add all of this to the oven to bake for some time. After 45 minutes, the dish should be done.

5. Take it out of the oven and allow it some time to cool down before you slice it into squares and serve.

CHAPTER 8: SNACKS AND APPETIZERS

ZUCCHINI HUMMUS

What's Inside:

- Salt
- Grated lemon zest (.5 tsp.)
- Chopped dill, fresh (1 tsp.)
- Tahini (1 Tbsp.)
- Olive oil (1 Tbsp.)
- Chopped zucchini (1)

How to Make This:

1. To start this recipe, bring out a food processor or a blender and set it all up.

2. When that is ready, add in the salt, lemon zest, dill, tahini, olive oil, and zucchini to the mix and blend.

3. When this is nice and smooth, you can pour the ingredients into a bowl and then serve when you are ready.

SALMON CANAPES

What's Inside:

- Sliced zucchini in 12 rounds (1)
- Salt
- Tarragon, chopped (1 tsp.)
- Orange zest, grated (1 tsp.)
- Plain yogurt (.25 c.)
- Canned salmon (4 oz.)

How to Make This:

1. For this recipe, take out a bowl before combining the tarragon, salt orange zest, yogurt, and salmon together well.

2. When this is ready, lay out the zucchini rounds on a flat surface. Add the salmon mixture on top of the zucchini rounds and enjoy it.

SWEET POTATO FRIES

What's Inside:

- Sliced sweet potato (1)
- Olive oil (1 Tbsp.)
- Salt (.5 tsp.)
- Ground cumin (1 tsp.)

How to Make This:

1. Turn on the oven and give it time to heat up to 450 degrees.

2. While the oven is heating up, take out a bowl so you can toss together the olive oil, salt, cumin, and the sweet potato sticks.

3. When those are combined together well, you can pour them out onto a baking sheet with a rim. Make sure that it is all in a single layer.

4. Add the baking sheet with all of the ingredients into the oven and let them bake. You will need to keep a spatula on hand to flip these around to cook evenly halfway through the process.

5. After 20 minutes or so, the sweet potato fries should be done. You can take them out of the oven before serving.

MASHED POTATOES

What's Inside:

- Salt
- Butter (2 Tbsp.)
- Nonfat milk (.5 c.)
- Cubed and peeled russet potatoes (2)

How to Make This:

1. When you are ready to start this, take out a pot and add the potatoes inside of it. Cover them with just enough water to get all around the potatoes.

2. Add the lid on the pot and then cook the potatoes on high heat for a bit, until the potatoes have time to become soft.

3. After about fifteen minutes of this, we can take the potatoes from the heat and drain out the water. Make sure the potatoes get back to the pot when you are done draining.

4. This is where we add in the salt, butter, and milk. Use a potato masher to mash everything together until smooth.

5. Take a test and see if there needs to be more seasoning before serving.

QUINOA PILAF

What's Inside:

- Salt (.5 tsp.)

- Chopped parsley (2 Tbsp.)

- Raisins (2 Tbsp.)

- Pine nuts (.25 c.)

- Vegetable broth (1 c.)

- Rinsed quinoa (.5 c.)

- Chopped and peeled carrots (1)

How to Make This:

1. To start, take out a pot and heat it over the stove. Add in the broth and the carrot and then cook. You will want to stir this as you go and wait a few minutes until the carrot has time to brown.

2. When this time is up, add in the quinoa and the rest of the broth. Reduce the heat a bit to a simmer and cover the pot to cook the quinoa.

3. It will take around 15 minutes for the quinoa to cook through. When this is done, add in the salt, parsley, raisins, and pine nuts before you serve and enjoy.

KALE SALAD

What's Inside:

- Salt
- Orange zest, grated (.5 tsp.)
- Chopped thyme (1 tsp.)
- Dijon mustard (1 tsp.)
- Plain yogurt (.25 c.)
- Chopped carrot (1)
- Chopped radishes (3)
- Chopped and steamed kale (2 c.)

How to Make This:

1. Take out a big bowl and toss the carrot, radishes, and kale inside of it.

2. In a second bowl, add in the salt, orange zest, dill, thyme, mustard, and yogurt.

3. Toss the dressing in with the salad and then serve right away.

PASTA SALAD

What's Inside:

- Creamed herbed dressing (1 recipe)
  Chopped basil (.25 c)

- Black olives, sliced (.25 c.)

- Canned chickpeas (.25 c.)

- Baby spinach (1 c.)

- Elbow macaroni (2 c.)

How to Make This:

1. Take out a big bowl and then toss together the basil, olives, chickpeas, spinach, and macaroni.

2. When this is done, add in some of the dressing, toss around, and serve right away.

COCONUT RICE PUDDING

What's Inside:

- Coconut milk (.5 c.)
- Milk (.25 c.)
- Ginger, ground (.5 tsp.)
- Vanilla pudding mix (1 oz.)
- Coconut, shredded (.25 c.)
- Brown rice, cooked (2 c.)
- Pear, grated (1)
- Honey (2 Tbsp.)
- Figs, dried (.25 c.)

How to Make This:

1. Bring out a pan and add in the honey, coconut milk, milk, and pear on medium heat. Let this mixture get to a boil and then take all of the ingredients from the heat.

2. When this is done, slowly add in the rice, ginger, coconut, and pudding mix into this pan.

3. Mix it well, and then set to the side for a bit. It will take around ten minutes to finish this up and cool down.

4. When that time is done, stir in the figs and then mix it around gently before serving and enjoying.

YUMMY VANILLA PARFAIT

What's Inside:

- Agave (4 tsp.)
- Vanilla milk (1 c.)
- Figs, sliced (2 c.)
- Salt
- Agave (2 Tbsp>)
- Chia seeds (.25 c.)
- Vanilla (1 tsp.)
- Yogurt, Greek (1 c.)
- Almonds, sliced (.25 c.)

How to Make This:

1. To start this recipe, take out a medium bowl and mix together the salt, vanilla, agave, yogurt, and milk until they are well combined together.

2. When that is done, whisk in the chia seeds. Set the bowl aside and let it rest for a bit. 25 minutes should be enough for this one.

3. When that time is up, cover up the bowl and set it into the fridge. Make sure to let it stay there overnight.

4. The next morning, mix in the toasted almonds, agave, and figs to the bowl. Layer the mixture into the serving glasses and enjoy right away.

HEALTHY BISCOTTI

What's Inside:

- Splenda (.75 c)

- Coconut flour (1.5 c.)

- Sweetened coconut, flaked (1 c.)

- Vanilla (1 tsp.)

- Baking powder (.75 tsp.)

- Egg whites (2)

- Baking soda (.25 tsp.)

How to Make This:

1. To start this recipe, turn on the oven and let it heat up to 300 degrees.

2. While the oven is warming up, take out a bowl and mix in all of the ingredients inside. Use an electric mixer to help form this into a smooth dough.

3. Knead the dough and then turn it into 3-inch rolls with this dough. Take out a baking sheet and line with parchment paper before placing the rolls on top.

4. Press down on the rolls a bit and then add the whole pan to the oven. These can bake for a little bit.

5. After 40 minutes, the dough should be done. You can take them out and allow them to cool down. Slice them diagonally before adding them back into the oven.

6. After another 20 minutes, take these out, give them some time to cool down, and then serve.

NUT BAG

What's Inside:

- Salt (1 tsp.)
- Olive oil (1 tsp.)
- Brazil nuts (1 oz.)
- Almonds (1 oz.)

How to Make This:

1. Turn on the oven and let it heat up to 365 degrees. While the oven is warming up, crush both the Brazil nuts and the almonds gently before sprinkling on some salt.

2. When the oven is ready, take the nuts and add to a tray, stirring around in some olive oil at the same time.

3. Add the tray into the oven and then cook for a bit. After 8 minutes, the nuts should be done,5, and you can take them out of the oven.

4. Allow these to chill until they get to room temperature and then move to a paper bag before serving.

CHAPTER 9: LUNCHES ON THE GO

BAKED TILAPIA

What's Inside:

- Dried basil
- Thyme, dried
- Olive oil as a spray
- Salt
- Fillets of tilapia (2)
- Oregano, dried)

How to Make This:

1. Turn on the oven and set the oven so that it warms up to 350 degrees. While the oven is warming up, you can take out a baking sheet and line it with some foil and a bit of olive oil.

2. Arrange the fish on the baking sheet and then top with the olive oil, salt, and herbs.

3. Add the baking sheet to the oven and allow it to bake for a bit. After 15 minutes of baking, the fish should be done.

4. Take it out of the oven and allow some time to cool before we serve.

CRAB CAKES

What's Inside:

- Tartar sauce (.25 c.)
- Olive oil (1 Tbsp.)
- Crabmeat (2 c.)
- Salt
- Grated lemon zest (1 tsp.)
- Chopped dill (1 Tbsp.)
- Plain yogurt (.25 c.)
- Baby shrimp, cooked (1 c.)

How to Make This:

1. To start this recipe, we want to bring out our food processor or a blender. Use this to help us combine together the salt, lemon zest, dill, yogurt, and shrimp.

2. When this is combined, we can spoon it into a medium bowl. Then it is time to slowly fold in the crabmeat until it is well combined.

3. Form this mixture into four patties and then set to the side for a moment.

4. Bring out a skillet and heat it up on the stove. When the skillet is warm, add in the patties and cook until these are browned.

5. After about 5 minutes on each side, you should see that the patties are browned and done. You can serve them with the tartar sauce on top and enjoy.

VEGGIE AND HALIBUT PACKETS

What's Inside:

- Butter (2 Tbsp.)
- Salt
- Dried dill (1 tsp.)
- Grated lemon zest (1 tsp.)
- Halved halibut (6 oz.)
- Sliced zucchini (1)

How to Make This:

1. Turn on the oven and let it heat up to 350 degrees. While the oven is getting nice and warm, place two squares of parchment paper onto a baking sheet with a rim.

2. Take your zucchini and divide it up between the squares. Top each of these with a piece of halibut and then sprinkle each with half the dill, salt, and the lemon zest. Add on a pat of the butter to each one as well.

3. When this is done, you can fold the squares around the ingredients to make a packet and then seal the edges with some narrow folds. Add this to the oven to bake.

4. After about 20 minutes the halibut is going to be nice and flaky, this is a sign that it is done and you can take out to cool down before serving.

SWEET QUINOA SALAD

What's Inside:

- Ground pepper (.25 tsp.)
- Cinnamon (.25 tsp.)
- Salt (.5 tsp.)
- Juiced lemon (.5)
- Avocado oil (2 Tbsp.)
- A handful of sprouts (1)
- Toasted and crushed walnuts (2 Tbsp.)
- Raisins (2 Tbsp.)
- Diced apples (2)
- Sliced shallot (1)
- Cooked quinoa (1 c.)
- Chopped spinach (3 c.)

How to Make This:

1. To start this recipe, take out a big bowl and toss together the sprouts, walnuts, raisins, apples, shallots, quinoa, and spinach.

2. You can then drizzle on top of the oil and the lemon juice. Make sure to season with the pepper, cinnamon, and salt as well.

3. Toss all of these together to combine well and then serve.

VEGGIE RAMEN

What's Inside:

- Cilantro (1 Tbsp.)
- Boiling water (3 c.)
- Spiralized zucchini (.5)
- Spinach (.5 c.)
- Sliced mushrooms (4)
- Spiralized carrot (1)
- Sliced broccoli (.25 head)
- Sliced bell pepper (.5)
- Juiced lime (.5)
- Tamari (1 Tbsp.)
- Minced ginger piece (1 inch)
- Miso paste (1 Tbsp.)

How to Make This:

1. To get started on this recipe, take out a big bowl with a lid and add in the zucchini, spinach, mushrooms, carrot, broccoli, bell pepper, lime juice, tamari, ginger, and miso.

2. Boil the water up until it is bubbling and then add it into the pot with the other ingredients that you are working with.

3. Stir the ingredients around a few times to mix, and then add the lid on top of it all. Set it to the side for a bit.

4. After about 5 minutes, this should be done. You can take the lid off and garnish with some of the cilantro before pouring into your bowls and serving warm.

SWEET POTATO NACHO BOATS

What's Inside:

- Diced avocado (.5)
- Diced shallot (1)
- Diced tomato (1)
- Sliced black olives (4)
- Spinach (1 c.)
- Diced tempeh (.75 c.)
- Cayenne pepper (.5 tsp.)
- Apple cider vinegar (.5 Tbsp.)
- Coconut aminos (.5 tsp.)
- Balsamic vinegar (.5 Tbsp.)
- Sweet potatoes (2)
- *Cheese Sauce*
- Chili powder (.5 tsp.)
- Tahini (1 tsp.)
- Lemon juice (1 Tbsp.)
- White miso (1 Tbsp.)
- Cayenne pepper (.25 tsp.)
- Minced garlic clove (1)
- Vegetable broth (.5 c.)
- Nutritional yeast (.5 c.)

- Steamed cauliflower (.25 head)

How to Make This:

1. Turn on the oven and give it time to heat up to 400 degrees. While the oven is heating up, take out a baking tray and line it with some parchment paper.

2. Pierce your sweet potatoes using a fork a few times and then add to the prepared tray. Bake this in the oven for a bit.

3. After 30 minutes, the potatoes will be done. In the meantime, you can work with the cheese sauce.

4. To do this, take all of the ingredients for the cheese sauce and add them to a blender or food processing. Mix until they are nice and smooth and then set to the side.

5. Bring out a small skillet and heat it up over some medium heat. When this is warmed up, add in the cayenne, apple cider vinegar, coconut aminos, and balsamic vinegar inside.

6. Let these ingredients heat up for about three minutes at this time before adding in the tempeh. Make sure to toss around a bit as you are cooking these together.

7. After five more minutes, your tempeh should be nice and warm, and the sauce you are using should reduce a bit.

8. This is when we can cut open our sweet potatoes and add in the avocado, shallot, tomato, olives, tempeh, and spinach inside. Drizzle some of your

cheese sauce on top of it all and then serve these warm.

EASY TUNA MELTS

What's Inside:

- Cheddar cheese, grated (.5 c.)
- Sandwich bread toasted and gluten-free (2 slices)
- Salt (.5 tsp.)
- Plain yogurt (3 Tbsp.)
- Drained tuna (6 oz.)

How to Make This:

1. Turn on the oven so that the broiler has time to warm up.

2. While the oven is warming up, bring out a bowl and combine together the salt, the yogurt, and the tuna.

3. Add your toasted and prepared bread to a baking sheet with a rim. Spread each of the slices with half of your tuna mixture. Top it all with the cheddar cheese.

4. Place the baking sheet into the oven and let it cook for a few minutes. After three minutes, take the melts out, and then serve.

CHICKEN NOODLE SOUP

What's Inside:

- Rotisserie chicken meat (8 oz.)
- Gluten-free spaghetti (1 oz.)
- Salt (1 tsp.)
- Dried thyme (1 tsp.)
- Poultry broth (8 c.)
- Chopped celery (1)
- Peeled and chopped carrot (1)
- Leek (1)
- Olive oil (1 Tbsp.)

How to Make This:

1. To start, you can heat up a large pot over the heat until it is warm. Then add in the celery, carrot, and leek.

2. Cook this and stir it around on occasion until you notice the vegetables are starting to brown a little bit. This will take around five minutes.

3. When this is done, it is time to add in the salt, thyme, and broth. Bring these ingredients to a boil and then add in the noodles.

4. Stir these but let them cook until the noodles are nice and soft. After nine minutes of this, add in the chicken and let it cook for a bit longer.

5. Another five minutes will pass, and then you can serve the soup nice and warm.

BAKED CHICKEN TENDERS

What's Inside:

- Chicken breast sliced (6 oz.)
- Eggs (2)
- Ground mustard (.5 tsp.)
- Salt (.75 tsp.)
- Dried thyme (2 tsp.)
- Dried oregano (1 Tbsp.)
- Breadcrumbs (1 c.)

How to Make This:

1. Turn on the oven and give it time to heat up to 425 degrees. While the oven is warming up, you can bring out a rimmed baking sheet and get it all prepared.

2. Then take out a bowl and mix together the mustard, salt, thyme, oregano, and breadcrumbs with one another.

3. In a second bowl, you can add in the eggs and beat them a bit.

4. When you are done slicing the chicken strips, you can take them and dump them into the egg mixture and then into the breadcrumb mixture, making sure to tap off any of the excess coatings.

5. Add the chicken tenders onto the prepared baking sheet, keeping them in one layer along the way. Add into the oven to bake.

6. After 20 minutes, the chicken tenders should be done. You can take them out of the oven and allow them some time to cool down before serving.

TURKEY BURGERS

What's Inside:

- Healthy burger sauce (4 tbsp.)
- Hamburger buns (2)
- Salt (.5 tsp.)
- Sugar (2 tsp.)
- Fish sauce (.5 tsp.)
- Ground turkey breasts (6 oz.)

How to Make This:

1. Take out a bowl and combine the salt, sugar, fish sauce, and turkey breasts. Mix this well and then form the whole thing into two patties. Set aside for now.

2. When you are ready, heat up a big skillet over medium heat. When the skillet has time to heat up, add in the turkey burgers and cook until they are browned on both sides. This can take about six minutes total to get done.

3. After this is done, you can spread each bun with some of the sauce and then top with the turkey burgers that you just made before serving.

TURKEY MEATBALLS

What's Inside:

- Salt (.5 tsp.)

- Ground mustard (1 tsp.)

- Grated ginger (1 Tbsp.)

- Chopped cilantro (.25 c)

- Ground turkey breast (6 oz.)

- Nonfat milk (.5 c.)

- Gluten-free breadcrumbs (.5 c.)

How to Make This:

1. To start this recipe and turn on the oven to 375 degrees. Take out a baking sheet and prepare it with some parchment paper while the oven is heating up.

2. While the oven is warming, take out a bowl and then combine together the milk and the breadcrumbs and let this soak for a few minutes.

3. In another bowl, you can combine together the mixture of breadcrumbs, salt, mustard, ginger, cilantro, and turkey breasts. Combine this well, but do not overwork it too much.

4. Roll the mixture into 12 meatballs and then place them on the baking sheet that you already prepared.

5. Add the meatballs to the oven to bake until they are cooked through, which can take about 20 minutes to accomplish. Allow them some time to cool down before serving.

BEEF AND VEGETABLE SOUP

What's Inside:

- Salt (.5 tsp.)

- Dried thyme (1 tsp.)

- Poultry broth (7 c.)

- Halved green beans (1 c.)

- Chopped and cored fennel bulb (1)

- Chopped and peeled carrot (1)

- Chopped and washed leek (1)

- Ground beef (8 oz.)

How to Make This:

1. To start this recipe, take out a large soup pot and add in the fennel, carrot, leek, and ground beef. Cook this, making sure to stir on occasion until the beef has time to brown, and all of your vegetables in the pot are nice and tender.

2. That above will take around five minutes, and then it is time to add in the salt, thyme, broth, and green beans. Bring this all to a simmer and then reduce the heat to a medium-high.

3. After this time, you can simmer this for a few more minutes to get everything nice and warm before serving.

SIRLOIN STEAK SALAD

What's Inside:

- Papaya vinaigrette (4 Tbsp.)
- Torn romaine lettuce (4 c.)
- Olive oil (1 Tbsp.)
- Sirloin steak (4 oz.)
- Salt
- Dried oregano (1 tsp.)
- Ground cumin (1 tsp.)

How to Make This:

1. Take out a small bowl, combine the salt, oregano, and cumin together. Use this mixture to season the steak on both sides.

2. Heat up a skillet on your stove and then add in the sirloin as well. this needs to cook until it reaches the desired doneness that you like.

3. When this is done, which takes around five minutes on the side, if you like medium rare, then you can take the sirloin from the heat.

4. Slice up the steak and then toss it together with the papaya vinaigrette and the lettuce before serving warm.

INSIDE OUT CABBAGE ROLLS

What's Inside:

- Brown rice, cooked (1 c.)
- Salt (.5 tsp.)
- Dried thyme (1 tsp.)
- Ground mustard (1 tsp.)
- Napa cabbage, chopped (2 c.)
- The green part of the leek (1)
- Ground beef (6 oz.)

How to Make This:

1. To start this recipe, take out a skillet and heat it up on a skillet. When the skillet is warm, you can add in the salt, thyme, mustard, cabbage, leek, and ground beef.

2. Cook these together, making sure to crumble up the ground beef with the help of a spoon, so it has time to get browned up nice. This can take five minutes or so depending on the heat.

3. When this is done, add in the rice to cook. Cook to heat the rice through all the way.

4. After four minutes, this should be done, and you can serve warm.

HAMBURGER STROGANOFF

What's Inside:

- Zucchinis turned into ribbons (2)
- Cornstarch (1 Tbsp.)
- Nonfat milk (1 c.)
- Poultry broth (2 c.)
- Salt
- Dried thyme (1 tsp.)
- The green part of the leek (1)
- Cremini mushrooms, sliced (1 c.)
- Ground beef (6 oz.)

How to Make This:

1. For this one, we need to take out a skillet and heat it up on the stove. When this is warm, add in the salt, thyme, mushrooms, and ground beef.

2. Cook these together, making sure to crumble up the ground beef with the help of a spoon, until the ground beef is nice and browned.

3. In a small bowl, whisk together the cornstarch, milk, and broth. You can then add this to the skillet that you are using, along with the zucchini noodles.

4. Cook all of these ingredients together until the sauce has some time to thicken. This takes another two minutes or so to complete.

5. When this is done, divide up among two plates and serve warm.

CHAPTER 10: DINNER RECIPES FOR EVERYONE IN THE FAMILY

TILAPIA WITH SALSA

What's Inside:

- Cantaloupe salsa (.5 c.)
- Salt (.5 tsp.)
- Dried cumin (.5 tsp.)
- Olive oil (1 Tbsp.)
- Tilapia fillets (2)

How to Make This:

1. To start this recipe, turn on the oven and give it some time to heat up to 425 degrees.

2. While the oven is getting nice and warm, add the fish fillets to your baking sheet. Brush some of the oil on top and then sprinkle the salt and cumin on top.

3. Place the fish into the oven and bake until it has time to flake. After 10 minutes, these should be done.

4. Take the fish out of the oven and give them time to cool down for a few minutes.

5. When you are ready to serve, add the fish onto a plate and then top with half of your salsa before serving.

SALMON WITH LENTILS

What's Inside:

- Chopped parsley for garnish (1 Tbsp.)
- Chopped dill (1 Tbsp.)
- Lentils drained and rinsed (1 c.)
- Peeled and chopped parsnip (1)
- Chopped and peeled parsnip (1)
- Chopped and peeled carrot (1)
- Salt
- Ground cumin (.5 tsp.)
- Salmon fillets (2)

How to Make This:

1. Turn on the oven and give it time to heat up to 400 degrees. While the oven is getting warm, you can take the salmon out and season with some of the salt and cumin.

2. Add the salmon to a prepared baking sheet and then add to the oven. After 15 minutes, the salmon should be cooked through, and you can take it out of the oven to cool down.

3. While that is baking, take out a skillet and give it time to heat up. Add in the parsnip and the carrot

and cook, making sure to stir on occasion until these are browned.

4. After five minutes of that cooking, you can add in the lentils and the rest of the salt. Cook this until it is heated through as well, which can take another four minutes.

5. Stir int h dill and then take the ingredients from the heat.

6. When the salmon has time to cool down, add the lentils to a place and then add the salmon on top. Garnish with the parsley and then enjoy it.

FISH TACOS

What's Inside:

- Guacamole (.5 c.0
- Chopped cilantro (.5 c.)
- Cheddar cheese, grated (1 c.)
- Salt
- Ground coriander (.5 tsp.)
- Ground cumin (1 tsp.)
  lime zest, grated (1 tsp.)
- Cod, skinned (8 oz.)
- Corn tortillas (4)

How to Make This:

1. Turn on the oven and let it heat up to 350 degrees. While that is warming up, take out some aluminum foil to wrap up the tortillas and add them into the oven. These need to go for 15 minutes to warm up.

2. While the tortillas are warming up, take out a big skillet and heat it all up. When the skillet is warm, add in the salt, coriander, cumin, lime zest, and cod.

3. Cook these until you can get the fish to turn firm and opaque. This can take up to five minutes to complete. Take off the heat when this happens.

4. When you are ready to assemble the tacos, you can divide up the code among the tortillas. Then top

with the guacamole, cilantro, and the cheddar before you enjoy it.

OVEN-BAKED CHICKEN

What's Inside:

- Chicken legs (4)
- Eggs (3)
- Salt (.75 tsp.)
- Dried thyme (1 Tbsp.)
- Breadcrumbs (1 c.)

How to Make This:

1. To start this recipe, turn on the oven and give it time to heat up to 350 degrees. Then you can line a baking sheet with some parchment paper and set it to the side.

2. Take out a bowl and mix together the salt, thyme, and breadcrumbs. Then in a second bowl, you can beat the eggs.

3. Then take your chicken legs and dip them into the eggs before dipping into the breadcrumb mixture, tapping off the coating that is extra.

4. Add these to the prepared baking sheet, but make sure that they are just in one single layer. Add this to the oven to bake.

5. After 30 minutes, you can turn the baking tray around and close the oven again. Allow them to cook for another half hour before serving.

TURKEY MEATLOAF MUFFINS

What's Inside:

- Salt (.75 tsp.)
- Dried thyme (1 Tbsp.)
- Dijon mustard (1 tsp.)
- Beaten egg (1)
  breadcrumbs (.75 c)
- Ground turkey (12 oz.)

How to Make This:

1. Turn on the oven and give it time to heat up to 350 degrees. Coat a muffin tin with some cooking spray while that heats up.

2. Take out a medium bowl, and add in all of the ingredients, take some time to combine the ingredients together.

3. Divide this mixture into four of the muffin cups and then add into the oven to bake.

4. After 20 minutes, these should be done. Take them out of the oven and allow them some time to cool down before serving.

TURKEY AND SPINACH ROLLATINI

What's Inside:

- Crumbled feta cheese (.25 c.)

- Grated lemon zest (1 tsp.)

- Thawed spinach (1 c.)

- Salt (.5 tsp.)

- Sliced turkey breast (12 oz.)

How to Make This:

1. To start this recipe, turn on the oven and give it time to heat up to 325 degrees. While the oven is heating up, take out a baking sheet and line it with some parchment paper.

2. Place the turkey onto the baking sheet and sprinkle a bit of salt on top. Then spread the spinach over the turkey and sprinkle with some feta and lemon zest.

3. We can then roll the turkey all the way up around the filling and secure it with either some toothpicks or butcher's twine.

4. Add this to the oven and give it time to cook inside the oven. This will take about 25 minutes to complete.

5. When this time is done, take the turkey out of the oven and slice it up before serving.

SOUR CREAM HALIBUT

What's Inside:

- Dried thyme (1 tsp.)

- Chopped parsley (1 Tbsp.)

- Chopped dill (1 Tbsp.)

- Sour cream (1 c.)

- Salt (.5 tsp.)

- Halibut fillets (4)

How to Make This:

1. Turn on the oven and give it time to heat up to 350 degrees. While that warms up, take out a rimmed baking sheet and add on some parchment paper.

2. Place the halibut fillets on the prepared baking sheet and then sprinkle with some salt.

3. In a bowl, you can mix together the sour cream, thyme, dill, and parsley. Add this mixture all on top of the halibut before adding it all into the oven to bake.

4. After 20 minutes, the fish should be done. Take it out of the oven to cool down before serving.

ROAST RIB OF BEEF

What's Inside:

- Sliced celery sticks
- Shallots, peeled and halved (4)
- Beef stock cubes (2)
- Beef ribs (3 lbs.)
- Parsnips, peeled and halved (6)
- Leeks small (5)
- Carrots, peeled and halved (6)
- Olive oil (1 Tbsp.)
- Sage leaves

How to Make This:

1. To start this recipe, turn on the oven and give it time to heat up to 400 degrees.

2. While that is warming up, take one of the beef cubes and mix it with one tablespoon of the oil. Rub this new paste into your beef.

3. Bring out a pan and grease it up a bit. Then add on the beef so that you can sear it before adding to a roasting pan.

4. In the same skillet, cook up your leaks until they become golden before placing all around the beef in the roasting pan.

5. Then use the same pan again to cook the parsnips and the carrots before transferring them over to the roasting pan as well.

6. Top the beef with some shallots, celery, and safe. When all of the ingredients are in the roasting pan, add them all into the oven to bake.

7. After 45 minutes, the beef should be done. Take it out of the oven to cool down for a bit before serving.

FLANK STEAK AND CHIMICHURRI

What's Inside:

- Grated zest from half a lime
- Chopped cilantro (.25 c.)
- Chopped parsley (.5 c.)
- Olive oil (2 Tbsp.)
- Flank steak (12 oz.)
- Salt (.5 tsp.)
- Ground cumin (1 tsp.)
- Dried oregano (1 tsp.)

How to Make This:

1. Take out a bowl and use it to stir together some of the salt with the cumin and oregano. Use this mixture to sprinkle and season on top of your flank steak.

2. Bring out a skillet and then heat it up a little bit. When it is ready, add in the flank steak and cook this whole thing for a few minutes on each side.

3. Turn down the heat on the skillet, so it is on a low setting. You can continue to cook the flank steak until you get it to the desired doneness that you like. You need an internal temperature of 135 for medium-rare if that is what you like.

4. While the steak is cooking, take out your food processor or a blender and combine the rest of the

oil along with the rest of the slat, lime zest, cilantro, and parsley. Pulse these together about 20 times to combine them well.

5. When the flank steak is all done, you can slice it up nice and thin, going against the grain. Serve this with some of the chimichurri and enjoy it.

SHEPHERD'S PIE MUFFINS

What's Inside:

- Grated Cheddar cheese (.5 c.)
- Mashed potatoes (2 c.)
- Salt (.5 tsp.)
- Dried thyme (1 tp.)
- Green peas (1 c.)
- Chopped and peeled carrot (1)
- The green part of the leek (1)
- Ground lamb (6 oz.)

How to Make This:

1. Turn on the oven and give it some time for the broiler to reach a high temperature. While the oven is heating up, you can take out a skillet and get it heated up on the stove.

2. Add in the salt, thyme, peas, carrot, leek, and lamb into the skillet. Cook these, making sure to crumble up the lamb with a spoon until the lamb is all the way cooked, and the vegetables have time to turn soft and are done.

3. When you get to this point, take out a muffin tin and divide the meat mixture up among four of the cups. Top with some of the mashed potatoes and some of the cheese on top as well.

4. Add the muffin tins into the oven and allow them to broil long enough for the cheese to melt.

5. After three minutes in the broiler, take these out and serve nice and warm.

LAMB CHOPS

What's Inside:

- Lamb loin chops (4)
- Salt (.5 tsp.)
- Fresh parsley (.25 c.)
- Oregano leaves (.25 c.)
- Rosemary leaves (.25 c.)
- Dijon mustard (1 tsp.)
- Butter (1 Tbsp.)
- Breadcrumbs (.75 c.)

How to Make This:

1. Turn on the oven and let it heat up to 325 degrees. While the oven is getting warm, bring out a blender and combine together the salt, parsley, oregano, rosemary, mustard, butter, and breadcrumbs.

2. Pulse these ingredients together 20 times, or until everything is pulsed and well combined with the breadcrumbs.

3. Spread this mixture all over the lamb chops, making sure to press it down to get it to stick on the top of the meat.

4. Then take out a skillet and add in the lamb chops to that. Brown these for just a few minutes on each side before moving to your rimmed baking sheet.

5. Add the baking sheet to the oven and allow it some time to bake. When six minutes have passed, you can take the lamb out and give it some time to cool down before serving.

STUFFED BURGERS

What's Inside:

- Burger sauce (4 Tbsp.)
- Toasted bread (4 slices)
- Chopped basil (4 Tbsp.)
- Cheddar cheese, grated (.5 c.)
- Fish sauce (.5 tsp.)
- Dijon mustard (1 tsp.)
- Salt (.5 tsp.)
- Ground beef (1 lb.)
- Breadcrumbs (.25 c.)
- Nonfat milk (.5 c.)

How to Make This:

1. Take out a bowl and combine together the breadcrumbs and the milk. Allow these to rest together for 10 minutes.

2. In another bowl, combine the fish sauce, the mustard, salt, breadcrumb mixture, and the beef together and mix them together well.

3. Roll this mixture into eight balls and then pat each one out into a patty.

4. In another bowl, you can mix together the basil and the cheese. Sprinkle this on each of the patties and then top with another patty. Make sure to pinch the edges together to seal it.

5. Take out a skillet and preheat it on the stove. Place the burger patties into the skillet and heat them up so they get cooked through. This can take about five minutes on each side.

6. Serve these patties when they are done on the bread that you toasted and with about a tablespoon of the burger sauce over each one.

CHAPTER 11: FINISHING IT OFF WITH DESSERT

DEVILED EGGS

What's Inside:

- Salt (.25 tsp.)
- Chopped dill fresh (1 Tbsp.)
- Dijon mustard (1 tsp.)
- Plain yogurt, nonfat (.25 c.)
- Eggs (4)

How to Make This:

1. Take out a medium saucepan and add the eggs inside. Cover these with some water, making sure it is at least one-inch high.

2. Bring this water to a boil on the stove and when it starts to boil and bubble, take the pot off the heat right away and add the lid on top.

3. Allow your eggs to sit in the water for a little bit. After 14 minutes have passed, turn on some running water and add the eggs underneath to peel.

4. When the peels are gone, slice these up going lengthwise and then slowly spoon out the yolks. Put the yolks into a small bowl and arrange the whites on a plate, making sure that the cut side is the part that is up.

5. When this is done, add in the yogurt, salt, dill, and mustard to the yolk. Blend this with a fork to make it smooth and then spoon the yolk mixture back into the egg halves before serving.

SPICED WALNUTS

What's Inside:

- Shelled walnuts (24)

- Ground cloves (.25 tsp.)

- Ground ginger (.5 tsp.)

- Dark brown sugar (.25 c.)

- Butter (2 Tbsp.)

How to Make This:

1. Take out a skillet to start this one and melt the butter inside with the skillet on the stove.

2. When the butter is melted, you can add in the cloves, ginger, and brown sugar. Cook this, making sure to stir along the way as it boils.

3. When this time is done, you can add in the walnuts and let them cook for a bit as well.

4. After 3 more minutes of cooking, take the walnuts off the heat and allow them some time to cool down before serving.

CINNAMON POPCORN

What's Inside:

- Butter, melted (2 Tbsp.)
- Popcorn, air-popped (6 c.)
- Sugar (.25 c.)

How to Make This:

1. Take out a small bowl and combine together the cinnamon and sugar really well.

2. When that is done, pop the popcorn until it is all done. Then add it to a really big bowl.

3. Toss in the sugar and cinnamon mixture along with the melted butter. Stir it all around to coat all of your popcorn with the cinnamon and the sugar and then serve right away.

BAKED CHIPS

What's Inside:

- Salt (.5 tsp.)

- Olive oil (1 Tbsp.)

- Sliced Yukon Gold potatoes (1)

How to Make This:

1. To start this recipe, turn on the oven and give it time to heat up to 400 degrees.

2. While the oven takes some time to heat up, bring out a bit bowl and then toss the slices of potatoes inside.

3. Mix in the salt and the oil, tossing everything around to make sure the potato slices are going to be covered all over.

4. When that is done, take out a baking sheet with a rim and then spread out your slices of potato in a single layer on it. Add to the oven to bake for a bit.

5. After about 15 minutes, the potato slices should be nice and crisp. Take them out and let them cool down before serving.

CARROT AND RAISIN SALAD

What's Inside:

- Ground cinnamon (.25 tsp.)
- Maple syrup (1 Tbsp.)
- Nonfat plain yogurt (2 Tbsp.)
- Peeled and grated carrots (3)

How to Make This:

1. Start this recipe out by taking the carrot and grating it. Set the grated carrot to the side.

2. Take out a bowl and mix together all of the ingredients, including the cinnamon, maple syrup, plain yogurt, raisins, and the grated carrots.

3. Mix these together well until they are combined and then serve.

CAROB AND PEANUT BUTTER BALLS

What's Inside:

- Salt
- Carob powder, unsweetened (1 Tbsp.)
- Confectioners' sugar (3 Tbsp.)
- Crunchy peanut butter (6 Tbsp.)

How to Make This:

1. Take out a medium bowl and combine the salt carob powder, confectioner's sugar, and peanut butter.

2. When those ingredients are combined, you can roll the mixture into six balls.

3. Put into the fridge to chill for a bit before serving.

YOGURT AND MELON ICE POPS

What's Inside:

- Maple syrup, pure (2 Tbsp.)
- Plain yogurt (1 c.)
- Honeydew balls (2 c.)

How to Make This:

1. Bring out a blender or a food processor and then combine together all of your ingredients. You will need to process these together until they can become smooth.

2. When this is done, bring out an ice pop mold that has at least four parts to it. Pour your mixture inside as evenly as possible.

3. Add these to the freezer and let them sit for 8 hours or more until they are nice and frozen. Serve when ready.

BANANA DESSERT

What's Inside:

- Sugar (3 Tbsp.)
- Banana (1)

How to Make This:

1. Turn on the broiler and give it some time to heat up to a high setting.

2. While the oven takes some time to heat up, take the banana and peel it. Then slice it in half going horizontally.

3. Cut each of the halves into half going lengthwise as well. then add these pieces onto a baking sheet that is rimmed, making sure the cut side is up.

4. When this is done, add some of the sugar over the bananas before putting the baking sheet into the oven to bake.

5. You will want to check on the bananas on a regular basis to make sure that they are not going to burn.

6. After about four to five minutes, the sugar should start to melt and brown. This is how we know the bananas are done.

7. Take them out of the oven and serve once they have some time to cool down.

ALMOND MERINGUE COOKIES

What's Inside:

- Sugar (.75 c.)
- Salt
- Cream of tartar (.25 tsp)
- Orange zest, grated (.25 tsp.)
- Almond extract (1 tsp.)
- Egg whites (2)

How to Make This:

1. Turn on the oven to start this recipe and give it some time to heat to 300 degrees. While the oven is getting warm, use some parchment paper to line the baking sheet and set this to the side.

2. When you are ready, bring out a large bowl and add in the salt, cream of tartar, orange zest, almond extract, and egg whites.

3. Take out your electric mixture and start beating these ingredients together, going on a high setting until the mixture starts to make some stiff peaks as well.

4. With the mixer still running, add in the sugar, going in a thin little stream until it has time to get into the bowl.

5. When this is done, spoon the meringue into 12 mounds on that baking sheet with the parchment paper.

6. Add the cookies into the oven and let them bake. You want to make sure that the cookies brown a bit and become crispy.

7. After 25 minutes, the cookies should be done. Take them out of the oven and give them some time to cool down before serving.

PEANUT BUTTER COOKIES

What's Inside:

- Egg (1)
- Brown sugar (1 c.)
- Peanut butter (1 c.)

How to Make This:

1. To start this recipe, turn on the oven and let it heat up to 350 degrees. While the oven is warming up, take out a baking sheet that you want to use and top it with some parchment paper.

2. You can then take out a medium bowl and add in the egg, brown sugar, and peanut butter of choice. Cream these together until you can get all of the ingredients to mix well.

3. After this, spoon the cookie batter into 6 portions onto that baking sheet, giving them some room to grow and expand.

4. Add the cookies into the oven to bake for a little bit. You want to allow the bottoms to have time to brown as well.

5. After about 6 to 8 minutes, the cookies should be done. Take them out of the oven and give them a bit of time to cool before serving.

BANANA PUDDING

What's Inside:

- Sliced and peeled banana (1)
- Vanilla (.5 tsp.)
- Nonfat milk (1 c.)
- Cornstarch (2 Tbsp.)
- Sugar (.25 c.)

How to Make This:

1. Bring out a smaller bowl to start and add in the cornstarch and the sugar. Make sure to mix around in order to combine.

2. Then it is time to bring out a small pan and add in the milk to it. Turn on the heat on the stove and let it simmer for a bit, stirring the whole time.

3. When the milk is nice and hot, pour your sugar and cornstarch mixture into this, making sure to whisk constantly the whole time.

4. Cook this for another 5 minutes, making sure to stir the mixture constantly the whole time. You know it is done when the mixture starts to coat the back of your spoon.

5. After this time, take the pan off the heat and whisk in your vanilla. Divide up the slices of banana that you did before among four ramekins.

6. Pour the pudding on top as evenly as you can. Then add to the fridge to cool down before you serve.

CHAPTER 12: VEGAN AND VEGETARIAN OPTIONS

POTATO SOUP MEDLEY

What's Inside:

- Chopped vegetables, raw (.5 lbs.)
- Fresh herbs
- Potatoes (.66 lbs.)
- Olive oil (1 Tbsp.)
- Vegetable stock (3 c.)

How to Make This:

1. Bring out a cooking pot and grease it up with some oil. Then add in the potatoes and the vegetables and cook until they are nice and soft.

2. When this is done, you can stir the stock into it and bring the mixture to a simmer to cook for a bit.

3. After 15 minutes, the soup should be done. Bring out the blender and blend the ingredients to make them smooth.

4. Serve this nice and warm with some fresh herbs to the top.

VEGAN SPAGHETTI

What's Inside:

- Peas, frozen (2 c.)

- Olive oil (2 Tbsp.)

- Egg whites (4)

- Whole meal spaghetti (3.25 c.)

- Hard cheese, vegetarian (.25 c.)

- Watercress (.25 c.)

How to Make This:

1. Start this recipe by heating water in a pot until it reaches the simmering point. Add in the peas here.

2. Cook these for just a couple of minutes before draining the peas and setting them to the side.

3. Blend these prepared peas with the cheese and the watercress until it is able to form a nice thick paste for you to use. Add in some olive oil and blend some more to make this all smooth.

4. At the same time, we are able to make spaghetti. Use the instructions on the package to boiling the noodles and then drain when it is done, setting the noodles aside until you are ready to use them.

5. Add water to your chosen cooking pot and bring it all to a simmer. When the simmer is reached, create a whirlpool in the water and add the egg whites. These need to cook for a few minutes as well.

6. Mix your pesto with the spaghetti and then serve with the watercress and the poached eggs on top before enjoying it.

EASY VEGETABLE SOUP

What's Inside:

- Worcestershire sauce (1 tsp.)
- Potato, chopped (1)
- Caraway seeds (1 Tbsp.)
- Sourdough bread, sliced (.5 lb.)
- White cabbage, shredded (.25 lb.)
- Cauliflower florets (.5 lb.)
- Bay leaves (2)
- Vegetable stock (3 c.)
- Chopped celery stick (1)
- Carrot, chopped (1)
- Rosemary sprigs (2)
- Olive oil (3 Tbsp.)
- Golden caster sugar (.25 tsp.)

How to Make This:

1. Turn on the oven and give it time to heat up to 320 degrees. When the oven is heating up, you can take out a baking tray and spread out the bread with the salt, caraway seeds, and one tablespoon of the oil. Add this to the oven to bake.

2. After ten minutes, the ingredients should be golden, and you can take them out of the oven.

3. At the same time, you can bring out a pot and add in the rest of the oil with the potato and the carrots. Cook for a bit to make these soft.

4. When that time is done, which will take around 5 minutes, stir in the rosemary thyme, bay leaves, stock, sugar, seasoning, and celery.

5. Boil this mixture, and when it reaches to that, reduce the heat to a simmer. Cook for a bit longer.

6. After another ten minutes is done, add in the cabbage along with the cauliflower and cook for a bit longer as well.

7. After 15 minutes, it should be done so you can stir in the Worcestershire sauce.

8. Discard the rosemary, thyme, and bay leaves and then serve this soup nice and warm.

LENTIL TACOS

What's Inside:

- Fresh cilantro, chopped (.25 c.)
- Avocado, chopped (.25)
- Salt
- Coriander, ground (.5 tsp.)
- Cumin, ground (1 tsp.)
- Vegetable broth (.25 c)
- Canned lentils (2 c.)
- Chopped and washed leek (1)
- Corn tortillas (4)

How to Make This:

1. To start this recipe, turn on the oven and let it have time to heat up to 350 degrees.

2. While that is heating up, take the tortillas and wrap them in some foil. Add them into the oven to warm for about 15 minutes.

3. During that time, we can bring out a big pan and add the leek. Cook the leek to make it soft.

4. After that time is up, add in the salt, coriander, cumin, vegetable broth, and lentils.

5. Bring all of these ingredients to a simmer and then lower the heat to get it to medium. Simmer it all, making sure to stir on occasion.

6. When you are ready to serve all of this, you can lay the tortillas out on a smooth surface and spoon the lentil mixture on top.

7. Top it all with the avocado and cilantro before serving.

CARROT AND ZUCCHINI FRITTATA

What's Inside:

- Salt
- Chopped thyme (1 Tbsp.)
- Eggs (4)
- Grated zucchini (1)
- Chopped carrot (1)

How to Make This:

1. Turn on the broiler and give it time to turn nice and warm.

2. In a big skillet, you can add in the carrot and cook it so it can become nice and soft. This takes around 3 or 4 minutes.

3. Add in the zucchini at this time and cook for a little bit longer.

4. While that is cooking, you can bring out a medium bowl and whisk the eggs along with the salt and the thyme.

5. Take your vegetables and spread them out as evenly as possible at the bottom of the skillet that you are using.

6. Slowly pour the eggs over these and lower the heat to a medium. We want to cook this, so the eggs have time to set around the edges.

7. Then use a spatula to help us pull the set parts of the egg away from the sides of the skillet. You can

also tilt the skillet to distribute the uncooked eggs into the space that you made.

8. We can continue to cook for a few more minutes until the egg is cooked and set on the edges.

9. When we get to this part, we are able to transfer the skillet over to our preheated broiler. Broil for a few minutes to get the top to set.

10. After about 3 minutes, we can take the frittata out of the oven and then cut into wedges to help serve.

TOFU RICE AND VEGETABLES

What's Inside:

- Miso paste (1 tsp.)

- Vegetable broth (.25 c.)

- Cooked brown rice (3 c.)

- Ginger, grated (1 Tbsp.)

- Chopped tofu (3 oz.)

- Broccoli florets (.5 c.)

- Chopped and peeled carrot (1)

- Chopped and washed leek, the green parts (1)

How to Make This:

1. Take out a skillet and heat it up on the stove. Add in the ginger, tofu, broccoli, carrot, and leek.

2. Cook these until the veggies are soft. This can take around five minutes. When this part is done, add in the rice to cook for a bit.

3. In a small bowl, we want to take some time to wish together the miso and the broth. Add this into the skillet with the rice.

4. Cook all of the ingredients and stir around to warm them up. After another 4 minutes, the dish should be done, and we can serve it.

CHEESE AND BROCCOLI BAKED POTATO

What's Inside:

- Cheddar cheese, grated (.5 c)
- Sea salt (.5 tsp.)
- Broccoli florets (1 c.)
- Russet potatoes (2)

How to Make This:

1. Turn on the oven and give it time to heat up to 350 degrees. While the oven is getting nice and warm, pierce the potatoes using a fork a few times.

2. Add the potatoes onto a baking sheet and add them to the oven. Let them bake for a bit.

3. After an hour has passed, you can take the potatoes out. Add the broccoli to the pan and keep it all in a single layer. Cook so the potatoes have time to get soft, and the broccoli can become tender.

4. After half an hour is done, take the potato and broccoli out of the oven. Let them cool down a bit before splitting open the potato.

5. Season with the salt before topping with both the cheddar and the broccoli. Server when ready.

PASTA WITH WALNUT PESTO

What's Inside:

- Cooked penne, gluten-free is the best (1 c.)
- Salt (.5 tsp.)
- Grated lemon zest (1 tsp.)
- Olive oil (1 Tbsp.)
- Parmesan cheese (.25 c.)
- Walnuts (.25 c.)
- Basil leaves, packed in tightly (.25 c.)

How to Make This:

1. To start this one, make sure to cook up the pasta noodles base don the instructions on the box. You want them to be al dente when they are done. Take out of the water, drain, and set aside for now.

2. Bring out your food processor or a blender and combine the salt, lemon zest, olive oil, Parmesan, walnuts, and basil inside.

3. Put the lid on top and then pulse these 15 to 20 times until it is well chopped. Toss this pesto with your cooked pasta and then serve.

CARROT AND ZUCCHINI FRITTATA

What's Inside:

- Salt (.25 tsp.)
- Chopped thyme (1 Tbsp.)
- Eggs (4)
- Grated zucchini (1)
- Chopped carrot (1)
- Olive oil (1 Tbsp.)

How to Make This:

1. Turn on your broiler to start this one and let it get to a high setting.

2. While the oven is heating up, take out one of your skillets and heat up the olive oil over a medium-high heat setting. Let the oil get to shimmering before continuing.

3. At this time, add in the carrots and cook, making sure to stir around. The carrot needs to start softening here.

4. After three minutes have passed, add in the zucchini and cook for another 2 minutes.

5. Take out another bowl and whisk together the eggs with your salt and the thyme.

6. Make sure to spread the vegetables out so that they are evenly on the bottom of the skillet. Pour the eggs on top of this and then lower the heat of the whole thing to medium.

7. Cook the egg mixture until it starts to set around the edges, which can take about 2 minutes.

8. Use your spatula in order to pull the set parts of the eggs away from the sides of your skillet. Then tilt it a bit in order to get the uncooked parts of the egg to end up in the new spaces you made.

9. Cook these eggs for another few minutes, so they have time to set around the edges again here.

10. When this is done, it is time to move the skillet over to the broiler. Broil these until the eggs have time to set on top.

11. After about three minutes in the broiler, take the eggs out and allow them time to cool down.

12. Slice the frittata into wedges and then serve.

ASIAN VEGGIE STIR-FRY

What's Inside:

- Bok choy, chopped (2 c.)
- Chopped and peeled carrots (2)
- Chopped and washed leek, only the green (1)
- Cubed tofu, firm (6 oz.)
- Olive oil (1 Tbsp.)
- Salt (.5 tsp.)
- Orange zest, grated (.5 tsp.)
- Grated ginger (.5 tsp.)
- Miso paste (1 tsp.)
- Vegetable broth (.25 c.)

How to Make This:

1. To start this recipe, bring out a bowl and whisk together the salt, orange zest, ginger, miso, and broth.

2. When that is done, set aside and then bring out a skillet. Add the olive oil to it and give the oil time to heat up until it starts to shimmer.

3. Add in the bok choy, carrots, leek, and tofu. Cook, making sure to stir on occasion here until the veggies have time to brown a little bit.

4. After five minutes of cooking the vegetables, you can add in the sauce that you set aside. Let it cook in the skillet until it has time to simmer.

5. Cook this and let the sauce have some time to thicken before you serve.

BROWN RICE LETTUCE WRAPS

What's Inside:

- Lettuce leaves, large (4)
- Chopped cilantro (2 Tbsp.)
- Salt (.5 tsp.)
- Vegetable broth (.25 c.)
- Ginger, grated (1 Tbsp.)
- Crunchy peanut butter (2 Tbsp.)
- Brown rice, cooked (1.5 c.)
- Firm tofu, cubed (3 oz.)
- Chopped and washed leek, just the green (1)
- Olive oil (1 Tbsp.)

How to Make This:

1. Bring out a skillet and add in the olive oil. You want to cook this until the oil starts to shimmer. When the oil gets to this point, you can add in the tofu and the leek and cook, stirring until the leek is nice and soft.

2. This takes around five minutes, so when that time is done, add in the salt, broth, ginger, peanut butter, and rice.

3. Cook these ingredients together, making sure to keep stirring so that it starts to get blended together well.

4. After four minutes of this, stir in the cilantro and mix together a little bit more.

5. Spoon this rice mixture into the lettuce leaves, roll them up, and then serve while nice and hot.

BUTTERNUT RISOTTO

What's Inside:

- Parmesan cheese, grated (.25 c.)
- Salt (.5 tsp.)
- Dried thyme (1 tsp.)
- Arborio rice (.5 c.)
- Butternut squash, cubed (1 .)
- Olive oil (1 Tbsp.)
- Vegetable broth (2 c.)

How to Make This:

1. Take out a saucepan that can fit quite a bit in it and then heats up the broth on the stove. Make sure to keep this one warm.

2. In another pan, heat up the olive oil on the stove as well, letting it go until it starts to shimmer a bit.

3. When the oil is shimmering, you can add in the squash and cook it. We want to get the squash to start to brown.

4. After four minutes of the squash cooking, add in the thyme and the rice and let it cook for a little bit more.

5. Using a ladle, add in the hot broth one bit at a time, making sure to stir on a consistent basis.

6. As you see, the rice starts to look a bit dry, add in some more of the broth, continuing this until the

broth has time to become nice and tender. This can take a bit of time, about 15 minutes to complete.

7. When this is done, turn off the heat. Stir in the Parmesan and the cheese to the mixture before serving.

EGGPLANT BURGERS

What's Inside:

- Lemon yogurt sauce (.25 c.)
- Hamburger buns, without any gluten (2)
- Eggplant slices 92)
- Salt (.5 tsp.)
- Dried oregano (1 tsp.)
- Ground cumin (1 tsp.)
- Olive oil (1 Tbsp.)

How to Make This:

1. Bring out your indoor or your outdoor grill and turn it on to high, so it has time to heat up.

2. While the grill is heating up, bring out a bowl and combine the salt, oregano, cumin, and olive oil together.

3. Brush the oil mixture on both sides of the slices of eggplant that you have. Then you can brush the rest of this mixture, if there is any, on the inside of your buns.

4. Add the eggplant slices to your grill and let them bake for a bit until they are brown. This can take up to 5 minutes on each side.

5. Add the buns to the grill and let them heat up to become toasted as well. This won't take too long to complete, usually about 60 seconds.

6. When the buns are done, it is time to assemble the burgers. Add the eggplant slices to the toasted buns and then top with some of the yogurt sauce before enjoying it.

FRIED EGG SANDWICH

What's Inside:

- Toasted gluten-free bread (2 slices)
- Salt
- Egg (1)
- Butter (3 tsp.)

How to Make This:

1. To start this recipe, bring out your skillet and heat up one of the teaspoons of butter until it has time to melt. You can swirl it all around the skillet to make sure that the whole thing is coated with butter.

2. When this is done, crack an egg into this butter and season it with some salt.

3. Cook until the egg is just setting, which can take about four minutes or so. Then it is time to flip the egg over.

4. When the egg has flipped, you can turn off the heat and allow it to sit there on the warm skillet for about 45 seconds to finish up.

5. Take out your toast and use the rest of the butter to spread on top of it. Slowly move the egg over to one of the slices of bread and then top with the other before serving.

CONCLUSION

Thank you for making it through to the end of *Acid Reflux Diet*, let's hope it was informative and able to provide you with all of the tools you need to achieve your goals whatever they may be.

The next step is to get started with the work we need to do with the Acid Reflux Diet. The longer that you let this go and do not take care of the problem, the worse it is going to get. You will find that starting on this diet and working to get your body back into shape and back into balance, the better that it can be for our whole health. Too often, we assume that the acid reflux is not that big of a deal and we are just fine with it. But in reality, we are missing out on so much of our good health when we rely on just using some over the counter medicines to heal it. Taking the time to really work with our health and deal with the acid reflux is going to be imperative to helping us get the best results.

And this is where this guidebook is going to come into play. It will help us to learn the right steps to take in order to get that acid reflux under control. We will first dive into what acid reflux is all about and why it matters so much to our health. Then we dive into some of the importance of why we need to worry about our pH levels and how the foods we consume are going to help to balance this out and get us in better health overall. And then we will end with a bit of information on the best recipes and meal plan that you can follow to get your health in line the way that you deserve.

You do not need to suffer from acid reflux for the rest of your life. There is so much more than you can work with and enjoy the process. This guidebook is going to walk you through some of that and help you to see how great it can be when you take control over your own health. When you are ready to learn more about acid reflux and how to put a stop to it before it causes more harm to your own body, make sure to check out this guidebook to help you get started.